THE VACCINE CRIME REPORT

MUST READ BEFORE YOU DECIDE TO VACCINATE YOUR CHILD

Dr. Kamalpreet Singh

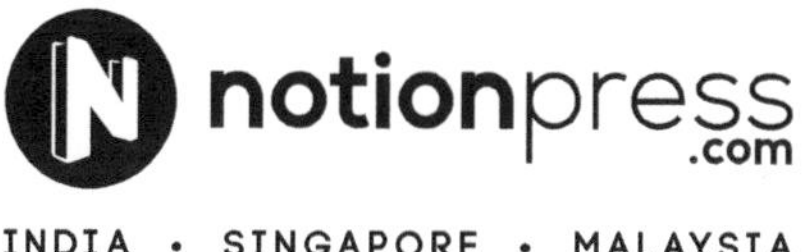

INDIA • SINGAPORE • MALAYSIA

ISBN 979-8-88772-967-1

DEDICATION

This book is dedicated to the millions of children who have suffered vaccine-related injuries and to their families, who have endured unimaginable hardships. *The Vaccine Crime Report* exposes the alarming correlation between the dramatic increase in childhood vaccine doses and the rise in autism, autoimmune diseases, chronic neurological disorders, reproductive issues, and other debilitating illnesses. Backed by scientific evidence, this book dismantles the misleading public narrative that vaccines are universally safe and effective. I offer my sincere gratitude to the Almighty for blessing me with strength, courage, and perseverance to walk the path of Truth, Freedom, and Health.

DISCLAIMER

The text, graphics, images, and other materials in this book are provided for informational purposes only. They are not intended to replace professional medical advice, diagnosis, or treatment. Always consult your physician or a qualified healthcare provider with any questions regarding a medical condition, treatment, or before starting a new healthcare regimen. Never disregard professional medical advice or delay seeking it based on information presented in this book.

PREFACE

The science surrounding vaccines is far from settled. Despite the prevailing narrative perpetuated by the media, the pharmaceutical industry, and much of the medical community, a substantial body of scientific evidence challenges these claims. This book is the result of an extensive effort to compile, organize, and present that evidence in a clear and accessible manner—so that every individual can evaluate the truth for themselves.

We are facing an alarming global health crisis. Over the past few decades, there has been an unprecedented rise in autism, developmental disorders, learning disabilities, allergies, asthma, and autoimmune diseases such as type 1 diabetes. Tragically, a significant portion of the next generation is lost to neurological, behavioral, and cognitive impairments. The statistics are deeply concerning. According to the Centers for Disease Control and Prevention (CDC), as of 2008, 1 in 6 children were diagnosed with either autism or some form of developmental disorder. Compare this to historical estimates: autism affected roughly 1 in 10,000 children in the 1950s, 1 in 5,000 in the 1970s, and 1 in 300 by the 1990s. If this trend continues, projections suggest that by 2032, 1 in every 2 children could be affected by autism. Additionally, rates of allergies, asthma, and autoimmune conditions continue to escalate at an alarming rate. This is a crisis we cannot ignore.

The vaccine debate is clouded by misinformation, bias, and assumptions—often originating from the very institutions people trust. *The Vaccine Crime Report* brings together a vast collection of credible scientific studies that challenge mainstream vaccine claims. Compiling this research has been an arduous yet necessary task, driven by my deep commitment to public health, particularly the well-being of children. As a healthcare professional, I have witnessed firsthand the devastating impact of developmental disorders, including autism, on families. These families are innocent victims in a system that prioritizes profit and control over health and safety.

The financial incentives behind vaccination programs are undeniable. The industry is a multi-billion-dollar enterprise, and those who promote vaccines often have vested interests in maintaining this revenue stream.

Conversely, those who raise questions about vaccine safety and efficacy do so at great personal and professional risk. Yet, open debate and healthy skepticism are essential in any scientific discussion. Blindly accepting any medical intervention without questioning its safety, efficacy, and long-term consequences is not only unwise but dangerous. I encourage skepticism—not just of vaccines but of any institution, policy, or practice that demands unquestioning compliance. An intelligent, informed individual seeks out facts, weighs evidence, and makes decisions based on truth rather than convenience or coercion. Critical thinking is not an act of defiance, it is a fundamental right and responsibility.

After dedicating countless hours to vaccine research—analyzing thousands of studies, reading extensively, interviewing medical professionals, and meeting with families affected by vaccine injuries—I have reached my own conclusion: vaccines are neither as safe nor as effective as they are claimed to be. I have chosen not to take any vaccines myself. I did not vaccinate my children. My sister did not vaccinate her children. My brother-in-law and sister-in-law did not vaccinate their children. We are all happy with our decisions, especially to watch our children grow into healthy individuals. However, this is our personal stance, and it is not shared by the majority of medical professionals, journalists, or policymakers.

The Vaccine Crime Report does not seek to dictate what you should believe—it seeks to equip you with the information necessary to make an informed decision for yourself and your loved ones. The choice is yours.

ABOUT THE AUTHOR

Dr. Kamalpreet Singh is a leading diabetes reversal specialist, clinical researcher, and medical nutritionist with over five years of experience in type-2 diabetes remission. He has successfully assisted more than 100 individuals to reverse diabetes through evidence-based nutrition and metabolic health strategies.

Dr. Singh serves as a Clinical Researcher at the Hospital and Institute of Integrated Medical Sciences (HIIMS), where he pioneers plant-based disease reversal protocols and integrative nutrition therapies. His expertise is backed by multiple international certifications, including Plant-Based Nutrition from Cornell University, Diabetes Reversal Coaching from the Institute of Food and Nutrition Therapy, and Fitness Nutrition from the American Council on Exercise.

Recognized for his outstanding contributions to plant-based disease reversal, he is a Dietitian under the Indo-Vietnam Medical Board and an honorary doctorate recipient for his groundbreaking contributions to medical nutrition. He is a member of esteemed medical networks, including the Network of Influenza Care Experts and Wellness & Inflammatory Syndrome Experts.

Dr. Singh has authored eight peer-reviewed research articles on diabetes reversal in leading medical journals, including the International Journal of Disease Reversal and Prevention, the Journal of Science of Healing Outcomes, and Ayushdhara Academic Journal. He has also been awarded by the India Book of Records for an extraordinary track record in medical nutrition services. A prolific author, he has written five books, including Advanced Nutrition Therapy, Shocking Truth of Paracetamol, and POSH Way to Reverse Type 2 Diabetes. His insights into holistic healing have made him a sought-after lecturer and keynote speaker at international health conferences, medical seminars, and wellness workshops.

Dr. Singh is also an expert in fasting and detoxification, having personally undertaken extended fasting protocols, such as 40-day grain fasting, 30-day juice fasting, 18-day coconut water fasting, and 9-day water fasting. His deep personal experience in fasting and detoxification has further shaped his innovative approach to healing.

As the innovator of the Supervised Diabetes Reversal Coaching Program, he integrates Moderate Glycemic Load diet strategies and Insulin Sensitivity Optimization techniques to help individuals restore their metabolic health naturally. His insights have been featured in international media, where he continues to advocate for a nutrition-first approach to healthcare.

Through his groundbreaking research, clinical expertise, and writing, Dr. Kamalpreet Singh is on a mission to redefine the future of healthcare—where food is the key to healing, prevention is the priority, and chronic diseases are no longer a life sentence.

FOLLOW THE AUTHOR

Dr. Kamalpreet Singh
WhatsApp: +1 416 795 1002
Website: https://gosatvik.ca/
Email: kamalpreetsingh@gosatvik.ca
Telegram: https://t.me/gosatvik
Twitter: https://twitter.com/gosatvik
Instagram: https://www.instagram.com/gosatvik
YouTube: https://www.youtube.com/@drksinghkhalsa

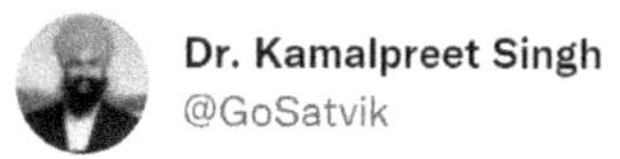

Dr. Kamalpreet Singh
@GoSatvik

Baby boomers had measles, mumps and chickenpox. Today's kids have autism, learning disorders, diabetes type-1, asthma, allergies, eczema, other autoimmune diseases, and even cancer. Isn't it the time to research, WHY??? What has changed?

4:21 PM · May 20, 2022 · Twitter for Android

7,568 Retweets **593** Quote Tweets **22K** Likes

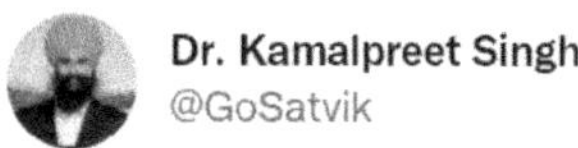

Dr. Kamalpreet Singh
@GoSatvik

If an unbiased and independent investigation of the vaccine industry is done - the ingredients, the health hazards, the money and parties involved, then one thing is for sure, the vaccines will go down as the most horrendous and hideous crime against humanity. Save the children!

7:32 PM · Apr 25, 2022 · Twitter Web App

Dr. Kamalpreet Singh
@GoSatvik

"The government is introducing mandatory weightlifting and sports, mandatory raw fruits and vegetables, mandatory sunbathing, grounding and deep breathing; while banning drugs, drinking and smoking." Have you ever heard your health minister say this? Is it really about health?

2:50 PM · Apr 13, 2022 · Twitter for Android

IMPORTANT STATEMENTS ON VACCINES MADE BY LEADING MEDICAL DOCTORS AND SCIENTISTS

"Vaccines are the backbone of the entire Pharmaceutical Industry. If they can make these children sick from a very early age, they become customers for life. The money isn't really to be made in the vaccine industry. The money is made by Big Pharma with all of the drugs that are given to treat and address all of the illnesses that are subsequent to the side effects of vaccines."

- Dr. Sherri Tenpenny D.O.

"I was involved in misleading millions of people about the possible negative side effects of vaccines. We lied about the scientific findings."

- William W. Thompson PhD
Senior Scientist CDC

"The vaccination process, by its very nature, entails significant risks of illness, injury, and death, which are persistently denied and covered up by the manufacturers, the CDC and the doctors who speak out in favour."

- Dr. Richard Moskowitz MD

"Anyone who tells you vaccines are safe and effective is lying. My view is that vaccines are unsafe and worthless. I would not allow myself to be vaccinated again."

- Dr. Vernon Coleman MBChB
General Physician, UK

"100 years from now we will know that the biggest crime against humanity was vaccines."

- Dr. Guylaine Lanctot MD
Phlebologist, Canada

WORLD HEALTH ORGANISATION: LEAKED CONFESSIONS ON VACCINES

There was a secret meeting of vaccine specialists of the World Health Organization. These specialists met to express their concern about the deaths caused by vaccines and its long-term harmful effects. This information was not supposed to leak out, but an honest person who had access to the footage of the secret meeting made it public. The footage highlights how dangerous the vaccines are. Here is what they said among themselves:

"We cannot overemphasize the fact that we really don't have very good safety monitoring systems in many countries. We're not able to give clear cut answers when people ask questions about the deaths that have occurred due to a particular vaccine."

- Dr. Soumya Swaminathan
Chief Scientist, WHO

"We have a very wobbly health professional frontline that is starting to question vaccines and the safety of vaccines. In medical school you are lucky if you have a half day on vaccines, never mind keeping up to date with all this."

- Prof. Heidi Larson, WHO
Director of Vaccine Confidence Project

"The major health concerns which we are seeing are accusations of long-term effects."

- Dr. Martin Howell Friede, Coordinator,
Vaccine Research Initiative, WHO

"It is not unexpected if they multiply the incidence of adverse reactions that are associated with the antigen but may not have been detected through lack of statistical power in the original studies"

- Dr. Stephen Evans, WHO

TABLE OF CONTENTS

SECTION 1

SECTION 2

SECTION 3

SECTION 4

EXISTING PROBLEMS WITH THE MEDICAL SYSTEM: MEDICAL MISTAKES – LEADING CAUSE OF DEATH

The current medical system is far from being safe. Medical researchers have continued to highlight the lower safety of the medical profession. An important example is the number of people that die due to medical error in hospitals every year. In 1999, the prestigious Institute of Medicine, published a report titled 'To Err is Human'. Dr Lucian Leape MD, a Harvard pediatrician who is referred to as 'the Father of Patient Safety' was on the committee that wrote the report. The report was published in the Journal of the American Medical Association (JAMA) and shocked the medical world. It stated that 98,000 people die annually due to medical mistakes in hospitals.[1]

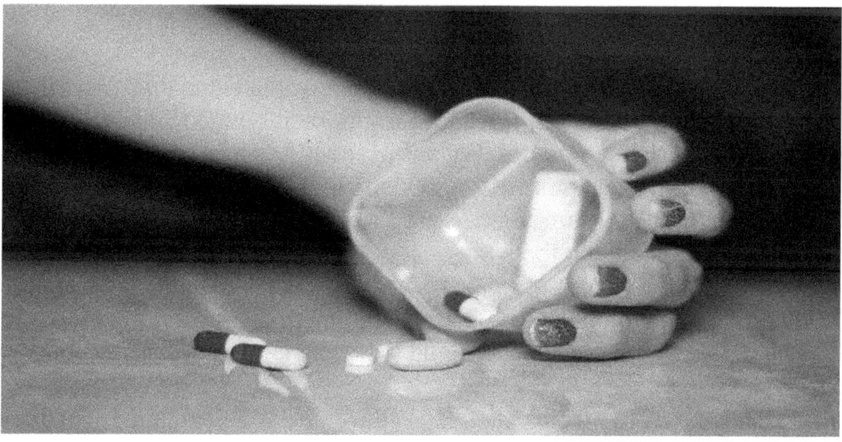

Another report titled 'Is US Health Really the Best in the World?' was published in Journal of the American Medical Association (JAMA) in July 2000 by Barbara Starfield MD. It states that the health care system contributes to poor health of Americans through its adverse effects. For example, every year United States estimates about 12000 deaths from unnecessary surgery, 7000 deaths from medication errors in hospitals, 20000 deaths from other errors in hospitals, 80000 deaths from nosocomial infections in hospitals and about 106000 deaths from adverse effects of medications. These total to 225000 deaths per year from iatrogenic causes which becomes the third leading cause of death in the United States, after deaths from heart disease and cancer.[2] Can you imagine that the medical system itself to be the third leading cause of death in the United States?

After a few years, a group of researchers thoroughly reviewed the statistical evidence and their findings on medical errors were shocking. Gary Null PhD authored a paper titled 'Death by Medicine' that presents powerful data that today's medical system often causes more harm than good. This fully referenced report demonstrates the number of people having in-hospital, adverse reactions to prescribed drugs to be 2.2 million per year. The number of unnecessary antibiotics prescribed annually for viral infections is 20 million per year. The number of unnecessary medical and surgical procedures performed annually is 7.5 million per year. The number of people exposed to unnecessary hospitalization annually is 8.9 million per year. The most stunning statistic, however, is that the total number of deaths caused by conventional medicine is an astounding 783,936 per year.[3] It might be somewhat correct to say that the medical system, itself, can be considered as the leading cause of death and injury in the United States. (It exceeds the number of deaths attributable to heart disease 699,697 and cancer 553,251 as per the statistics.)

Unfortunately, the news has continued to get worse since then. An article published in the Journal of Public Safety September 2013 titled, 'A New Evidence-based Estimate of Patient Harms Associated with Hospital Care', found that a minimum of 210,000 preventable deaths per year occur in the U.S. and that the number may exceed 400,000 because of the limitations of the search tools they used. Incredibly, they also determined that serious harm to patients in hospitals may be 10-20 times greater than that horrific lethal number of 400,000! That means between 4 million and 8 million people are seriously harmed in hospitals annually in the U.S![4]

According to a 2016 article published in the Journal of Community Hospital Internal Medicine Perspectives, titled the alarming reality of medication error: a patient case and review of Pennsylvania and National data, there is a dangerous and costly number of medication errors annually in the U.S. "Errors occurred at multiple care levels, including prescribing, initial pharmacy dispensation, hospitalization, and subsequent outpatient follow-up. This exemplifies the Swiss Cheese Model of how errors can occur within a system. Adverse drug events (ADEs) account for more than 3.5 million physician office visits and 1 million emergency department visits each year.[5] It is believed that preventable medication errors impact more than 7 million patients and cost almost $21 billion annually across all care settings. About 30% of hospitalized patients have at least one discrepancy on discharge medication reconciliation. Medication errors and ADEs are an underreported burden that adversely affects patients, providers, and the economy.

What do the above Statistics tell us?

This shows that medical industry has absolutely failed in the prevention and treatment of illness, sickness, and disease. More and more people are going to visit doctors than ever before. More and more people are getting diagnosed regularly through blood tests, X-rays, ultrasounds, etc. than ever before. More people are taking pills and drugs than ever before. There are more surgeries performed than ever before. But still, more people suffer from diseases like diabetes type-2, heart disease, hypertension, thyroid imbalance, polycystic ovarian syndrome, obesity, multiple sclerosis, asthma, bronchitis, sinusitis, chronic kidney disease, ulcers, piles, acid reflux, constipation, cancer, etc. The only winners in the medical system are the healthcare and drug companies. The drug companies' profits are skyrocketing. The medical industry has no genuine interest in the prevention and curing of any illness but their own profits.

In my personal experience with hundreds of people with the above conditions, I have seen that majority of these diseases that have been termed as incurable, are reversible and also curable within a few months by eliminating the cause of the disease by following a regimen of natural diet and lifestyle that has the potential to activate self-healing mechanism of the body. Anyone who is ready to eradicate the root cause of their disease will successfully recover if they un-do what caused the disease and start doing what heals it. You can read more about such natural cures in my book 'Advanced Nutrition Therapy: Goodbye Drugs and Diseases' or visit my website 'https://gosatvik.ca' to watch the testimonial videos of the patients healed through natural nutrition therapy.

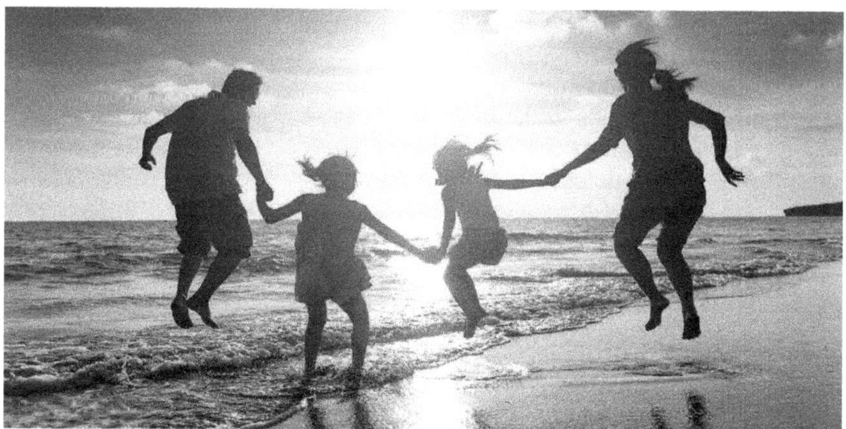

An ideal scenario would be waking up in the morning full of energy, vitality, content, and feeling blessed. You enjoy your day with energy, a bounce in your step, a smile on your face. You don't feel stressed, anxious, or depressed; you don't feel tired, you have no headaches or pain in your body; you are not overweight, and your skin is glowing. You have a good appetite and eat what you want, and you are never that hungry. You don't deprive yourself of the foods you enjoy. You go to sleep at night, and you sleep soundly and peacefully and get a wonderful whole night's rest. Your skin, your hair, and your nails look healthy and radiant. You have strength and tone in your muscles. Your body is fluid, graceful, and flexible. You are firm, strong, vibrant, and feel great! These are the signs of a healthy person.

A healthy person rarely needs to take a drug. A healthy person never has to have surgeries. Being sick is not "normal," it is abnormal. Most people think they are healthy, but they really have no idea just how much better they could feel. A healthy person has no cancer, diabetes, or heart disease. A healthy person lives without illness, sickness, or disease. Most people have no idea how good their body is designed to feel. We have been brainwashed into believing that it is natural for a human being to have aches and pains, and have major medical problems like cancer, diabetes, and heart disease. We are also brainwashed into believing that it's "natural" to take drugs. We are programmed to believe that we "need" drugs in order to be healthy.

Is there a place for surgery and drugs? The answer is absolutely yes! Medical science has done a decent job at addressing symptoms. However, the treatment of a symptom has two flaws. First, the treatment itself usually causes more problems which will have to be treated later. Second, the cause of the symptom is usually never addressed. When you do not address the cause, you are allowing for problems later on.

With this said, if you are in an emergency situation such as that caused by a sudden accident of some sort, drugs and surgery can save your life. However, drugs and surgery have failed at preventing illness and they do not address the cause of illness. Nevertheless, they do work well (not always) in most emergency crisis situations. The bottom line is, if you fall off a ladder and puncture an organ, you want to be rushed to the closest emergency room and have a trained medical doctor use drugs and surgery to save your life. But if you want to stay healthy and never have disease, drugs and surgery are not the answer. So, if trillions of dollars in scientific research have failed in producing ways to prevent and cure illness and disease, and all-natural inexpensive prevention methods and cures do exist, why aren't we hearing about them? The answer may surprise you.

What if the Cure is Discovered?

Imagine there is a scientist working in a lab somewhere.[6] He makes a breakthrough discovery: A small plant is found in the Amazon that, when made into a tea and consumed, eliminates all cancer in the body within one week. Imagine this researcher proclaiming that he has given this tea to one thousand cancer patients and that every single one of them, within one week and without having undergone surgery, was found to have absolutely no cancer in their body. Eureka! A cure for cancer! A simple, inexpensive, all-natural cure with no side effects. Just a simple plant that you make into a tea and drink. It has absolutely no side effects at all. It's pure, all-natural, and costs just pennies.

Imagine this scientist announcing his discovery to the world. Certainly, he would win a Nobel Prize. Certainly, the world medical community would be rejoicing. No more cancer! Every cancer patient could drink this tea and in one week be free of all their cancer. Every person who lives with the fear of getting cancer could now know that they could simply drink a few cups of this tea, which costs them only a few pennies, and they could avoid ever getting cancer. The world would be a better place.

Unfortunately, you'll never hear this story. Not because the story is not true, but because if this simple herbal tea which cures all cancer was allowed to be sold, there would be no need for the American Cancer Society. There would be no need for any of the drug companies that are manufacturing and selling cancer drugs. There would be no need for any additional cancer research funding. Cancer clinics around the world would close, hundreds of thousands of people would be put out of work, entire industries would shut down overnight and billions and billions and billions of dollars in profit would no longer be funneling into the kingpins who control the cancer industry.

So, when this person makes this discovery, what happens? In some cases, these people simply vanished. In other cases, these people were given hundreds of millions of dollars for their research. In still other cases the federal government raided these researchers' offices, confiscated the data, and jailed the researchers for practicing medicine without a license. Is this fantasy or is this the truth? Well, the health-care industry has a dirty little secret, and I am blowing the whistle on it.

You Must Judge: Is it Real Science or Tobacco Science?

In February 2006, the American Journal of Public health published an article titled, "The Doctor's Choice is America's Choice". This article chronicled the history of the cigarette industry's relationship with medical doctors. Medical doctors took center stage between 1930 to 1953 as the face of authority recommending cigarette smoking in tobacco company advertising. In the mid-1930s Phillip Morris, designed a campaign that referred directly to research conducted by physicians. The premise of their claim was based on studies showing that diethylene-glycol added to cigarettes made them "moister and less irritating" than other brands.[7] This "benefit" then appeared in various medical journals. This advertising touting medical doctors recommending various brands of cigarettes ran in those journals and became a steady source of income for well-respected medical journals including, the New England Journal of Medicine and the Journal of the American Medical Association.

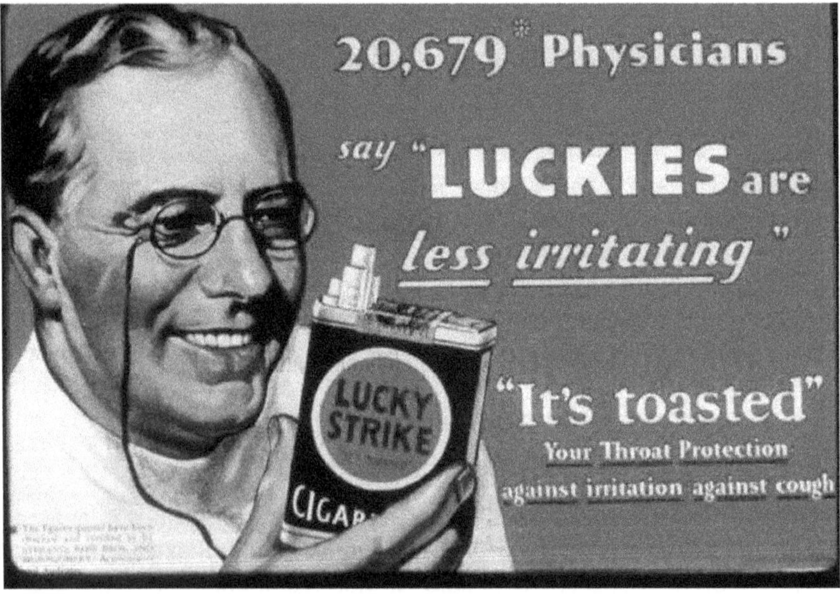

One advertisement by Lucky Strikes Tobacco bragged "20,679 physicians say, 'Lucky's are less irritating' and featured a white coated doctor with a reassuring smile. Can you imagine a medical doctor promoting the benefits of smoking cigarettes?

An Example of Medical Blunder that should Caution you:

Thalidomide was first marketed in 1957 in West Germany under the tradename Contergan. The German drug company Chemie Grünenthal developed and sold the drug. Primarily prescribed as a sedative or hypnotic, thalidomide also claimed to cure "anxiety, insomnia, gastritis, and tension". Afterwards, it was used against nausea and to alleviate morning sickness in pregnant women. Thalidomide became an over-the-counter drug in West Germany on October 1, 1957. Shortly after the drug was sold in West Germany, between 5,000 and 7,000 infants were born with phocomelia (malformation of the limbs). 40% of these children died.[8] Throughout the world, about 10,000 cases were reported of infants with phocomelia due to thalidomide: only about 50% of the 10,000 survived.

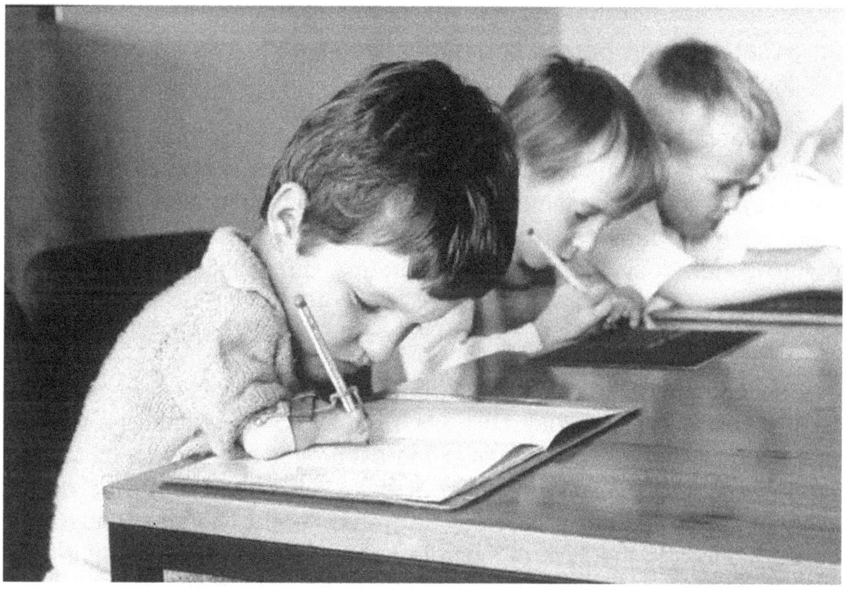

Those subjected to thalidomide while in the womb experienced limb deficiencies in a way that the long limbs either were not developed or presented themselves as stumps. Other effects included deformed eyes and hearts, deformed alimentary and urinary tracts, blindness, and deafness. This is important because if you are not cautious, you might end up taking experimental drugs, injections, therapies, or surgeries that might potentially turn your life upside down. The pregnant women who took Thalidomide had no idea that a fetal harming poison was being given to them in the name of medicine. The true results of the "medicine" came after some months when the limbs of their children were deformed.

Therefore, you must take the responsibility of your health and happiness in your hands. Do not blindly trust what is being told to you. Do not agree to any diagnostic system, medical procedure, or treatment unless you analyze the pros and cons yourself. Always ask the question: Will this medical procedure (drugs/surgery/injection/) improve my quality of life or life span as compared to not taking it? Study the evidence and then decide. It is important to be aware and awake to the reality. Always read the evidence before believing whatever is being propagated on television.

Always ask these Questions:

1. What does this person or organization stand to gain if I accept their claims?

2. What does this person or organization stand to lose if I don't accept their claims?

When I look at the groups and individuals that stand to gain the most by expansion of vaccination programs (Big Pharma, Legislators, Media, Doctors), it certainly becomes clear that money is the incentive that makes them push the agenda. Now, I will concede that there are some well-meaning individuals in each of those groups. But as I just mentioned, it is their responsibility to do their due diligence and stand up for truth in all appropriate ways.

The second group, i.e., vaccine skeptics, are the parents who are looking for the best interest of their child. And if they don't buy into the vaccine propaganda, then all those special interest groups also have a lot to lose! For families, there is so much more at stake in the health of their children. When you see vaccine injured children and the horrible and tragic consequences to the lives of those families, it is heart wrenching! It is an extremely difficult dilemma, so it's no wonder that so many are struggling over this issue.

WHY ARE VACCINES ASSUMED TO BE GOOD BY MOST PEOPLE?

It is because they are told that vaccines are "safe and effective." And who tells them? The trio of evil – government, pharmaceutical companies, and medical doctors. Drug companies make money out of vaccinations. And so do doctors. Politicians and government officials go along forth ride because they have been pressured into supporting vaccination by the drug companies and it becomes impossible for them to backout without exposing themselves to multi-billion-dollar lawsuits.

The few doctors who do stand up and dare to point out that vaccination programs are a hazard and do more harm than good, are quickly silenced. They are discredited, scorned, and their work is not published.

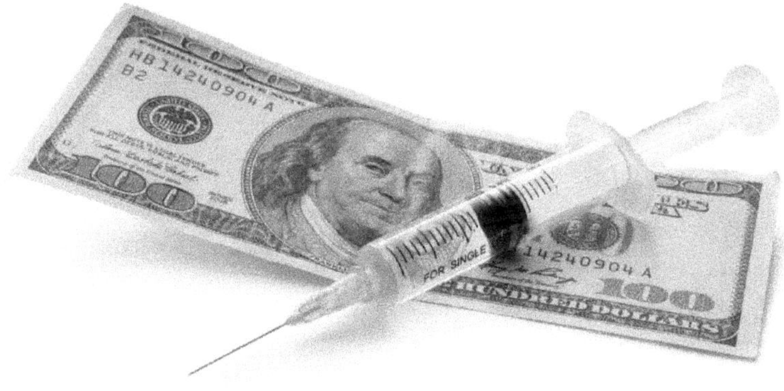

I have, over the years, discovered many of the hazards of telling the truth. Many organisations who initially promoted my work, started removing my content from their public displays. My social media accounts got deleted, banned or frozen multiple times. Even my WhatsApp account was blocked for spreading the truth during the Covid-19 plandemic.

Hundreds of medical doctors and scientists have been silenced, vilified, and humiliated for exposing the dark secrets of medical industry. I mention this to show that only one-sided information is provided for public consumption. The whole vaccination story is one of the great modern scandals of our time. It is astonishing that most doctors, whether working as hospital consultants, general physicians, or public health officials, know too little about vaccinations. Most of them simply follow what the medical establishment tells them. They never question what they are told by the drug industry and dismiss all critics of vaccination as dangerous lunatics and get extraordinarily rich by promoting mass vaccination programs which have never been proven to be safe or effective.

Over the years I have learned that the truth about many aspects of medicine is suppressed and, as a result, most people simply do not know the facts. The information generally available is provided by politicians, scientists and doctors who bend the truth for commercial reasons and then repeated by journalists who simply report what they are told.

The result is that millions of people make vital decisions based on half-truths and downright lies. Anyone who insists that vaccines are safe and effective is a liar, intentionally or unintentionally. Life is made easier for the liars because most people are overwhelmed with everyday life problems and readily accept what appears to be comfortable certainty. They want to trust advice from people they believe to be experts. All that makes the great betrayal even more shameful and unforgivable. Also, most general physicians fail to mention to the patients that they have a vested financial interest in promoting vaccinations.

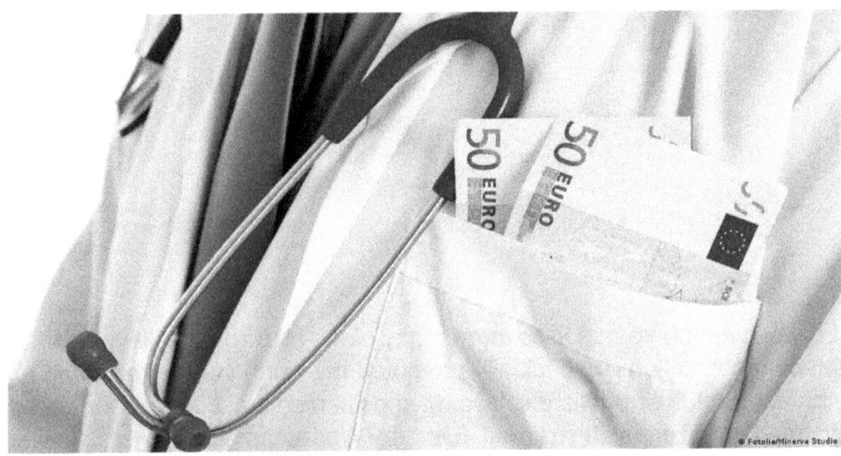

Most general physicians receive massive payments for giving vaccinations and huge bonus payments for vaccinating large quantities of their patients. A medical doctor who jabs enough patients gets a great amount of money straight into his bank account. A general physician who is questioning and discerning will be punished because he will not get the money. Drug companies and doctors make huge amounts of money out of this endeavour. Drug companies make billions. Doctors make thousands.[9]

Doctors are rewarded to maximize Immunization Compliance

Financial incentive often clouds judgement and reasoning. This image is just one example of how insurance plans incentivize doctors for immunization compliance.

CHILDHOOD IMMUNIZATIONS – COMBO 10	
Product lines	**BCN Commercial**
Source	HEDIS
Description	The percentage of children 2 years of age who meet the combination 10 criteria on or before their second birthday: • (4) DTaP* vaccinations • (3) IPV* vaccinations • (1) MMR vaccination • (1) VZV vaccination • (3) HiB* vaccinations • (3) Hepatitis B vaccinations • (4) PCV* vaccinations • (1) HepA vaccination • (2 or 3) RV* vaccinations • (2) Influenza** vaccinations *Vaccinations administered prior to 42 days after birth are not counted as a numerator hit. **Vaccinations administered prior to 180 days after birth are not counted as a numerator hit.
Continuous enrollment	Must be continuously enrolled 12 months prior to child's second birthday
Age criteria	Children who turn 2 years of age during 2016
Exclusionary criteria	Children who are documented with an anaphylactic reaction to the vaccine or its components
Numerator	The number of children who completed vaccinations as defined above
Denominator	The eligible population
Level of measure	Provider level
Target: COMM	63%
Payout: COMM	$400 per Combo 10 completed for each eligible member

You can see on page 16 of their 2016 plan booklet, that Blue Cross Blue Shield pays doctors $400 as an "incentive" (as they call it), for each "Combo 10" (which is a series of ten vaccines), that they provide children in their practice.[10] This of course is in addition to any other fees that the doctor collects for that office visit. At $400 per child, that adds up. By vaccinating only 100 children, the doctor pockets an additional $40,000 bonus. That is a good amount of money. Isn't that a conflict of interest?

Why would a medical doctor who can earn $40,000 by vaccinating 100 children sacrifice that amount and instead of that spend his time to research the truth of vaccine toxicity and raise awareness, and be vilified and inspected by their medical boards and colleagues? That is why it is not easy to stand up for truth and I have utmost respect for the honest doctors who do the right thing despite the challenges they have to face.

The Great Vaccination Myth: Should vaccines really get credit for the decline of infectious diseases?

Most practising doctors and nurses undoubtedly believe that vaccines have helped wipe out some of the deadliest infectious diseases. Many members of the medical profession would put vaccination high on any list of great medical discoveries. Those who promote vaccines often claim that vaccination programmes have reduced illness and prevented millions of deaths. These are all barefaced lies. This simply is not true; it is a myth.

The introduction of vaccination programmes came along either just at the same time or later when the death rates from the major infectious diseases had already fallen. The evidence shows that the diseases which are supposed to have been wiped out by vaccines were disappearing long before vaccines were introduced. It shows that vaccination programmes have not done the things they are credited with but have done most of the things they are blamed for.

The reason that most of these diseases were decreasing already was the significant improvements that were made in personal hygiene, improved sanitation habits, refrigeration, sewage elimination, better nutrition, and cleaner water supplies during the last hundred years. Improvements in trade and commerce also contributed to access to higher quality nutrition.

Anyone who doubts this has to only look at graphs showing mortality rates and life expectation rates alongside graphs showing when vaccines were introduced. The graphs show clearly that the improvements took place before the vaccines were introduced. Study the evidence related to whooping cough, tetanus, diphtheria, smallpox, and other diseases and it becomes clear that the incidence of these diseases, and number of deaths caused by them, were in decline long before the relevant vaccines were introduced.[11]

The graph on the next page depicts that the mortality for several common illnesses had already declined significantly long before the vaccines were created. The downward trend of the curves is completely unaffected by vaccine introduction.[12]

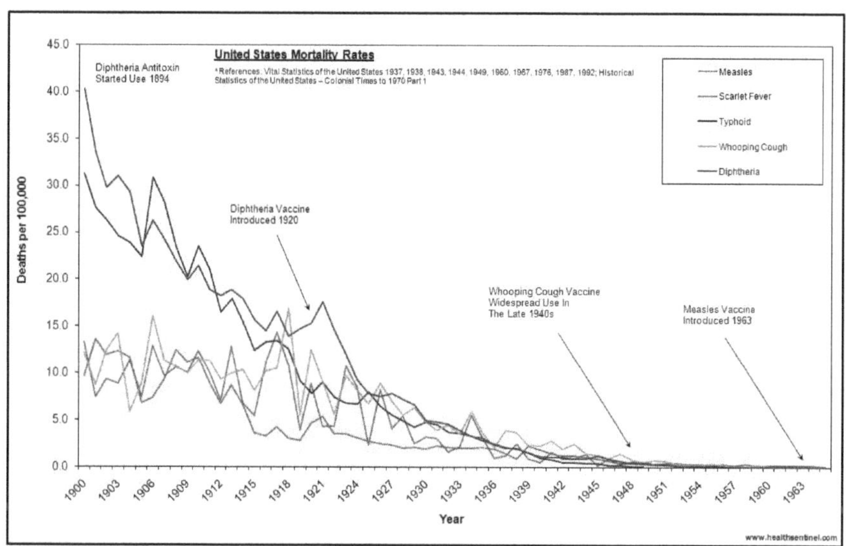

In recent history in underdeveloped and third-world nations, we have seen rates of infectious disease similar to what they used to be in western countries 100 years ago, prior to all these improvements. And yet, many of these impoverished nations are seeing dramatic improvements in hygiene, sanitation, better nutrition, and clean water. Also, the rates of infectious disease complications and deaths are also dropping significantly.

So, how do they fool the masses? A vaccine is introduced, and the trajectory of the disease goes down. The most important question that no one ever asks is, what was the trajectory of the disease before the vaccine was introduced? If the trajectory of disease was declining before the vaccine was introduced, it is probable that the vaccine got the credit for something it did not do.

The principle behind vaccination is a convincing one. The theory is that when an individual is given a vaccine - which consists of a weakened or dead version of the disease against which protection is required - his or her body will be tricked into developing antibodies to the disease in the same way that a body develops antibodies when it is exposed to the disease itself. But things aren't quite so simple. How long do the antibodies last? Do they always work? What about those individuals who do not produce antibodies at all? What about the adverse effects from the ingredients of the vaccine? What about the deaths and permanent disabilities caused to some of the vaccine recipients?

After spending countless hours on vaccine research: studying thousands of research papers, reading hundreds of books, watching dozens of censored documentaries, interviewing dozens of medical doctors, and meeting with children who suffered vaccine injuries, I concluded that vaccines are ineffective, unsafe and may cause serious health complications. I would not be taking any of the vaccines for myself. This is a personal view, and it is not a view shared by most doctors, nurses, and journalists. Those who are reading this book must make their own judgements and decisions based on all the available evidence.

The bottom line is that I do not advise anyone to not take a vaccine. I do not advise anyone to take a vaccine. I do not advise anyone to vaccinate or not vaccinate their child. My role, as a writer, is to provide information (which is not provided by the Government or the medical profession) and to give some idea of the sort of questions which readers may like to ask when considering a vaccination programme. So, before you allow your doctor to vaccinate your child you may ask him these essential questions:

1. How dangerous is the disease for which the vaccine is being given? How much probability exists that this disease can kill or cripple me?

2. Will you guarantee that this vaccine will prevent me from getting the disease? If not, what kind of protection is it supposed to give then?

3. Will you guarantee that this vaccine will not harm me in any form? If not, what are the adverse effects associated with it?

4. Will you take full responsibility for any adverse effect caused by this vaccine? If not, then how am I supposed to report the adverse effect and receive compensation?

5. Which patients should not be given the vaccine? Can you provide a list of all the ingredients in this particular vaccine?

Then ask him or her to sign a note confirming what he or she has told you regarding the above questions. If your doctor or nurse wants to vaccinate you, ask him or her to confirm in writing that the vaccine is both essential and safe. Ask your doctor or nurse to give you written confirmation that he or she has personally investigated the risk-benefit ratio of any vaccine they are recommending and that, having looked at all the evidence, they believe that the vaccine is safe and essential. How could any honest, caring, well-informed doctor or nurse object to signing such a confirmation.

Similarly, parents who are worried about having their children vaccinated should ask their doctor or nurse to sign a form taking legal responsibility for any adverse reaction. It is important to remember that most of the doctors (including nearly all GPs) who write and speak in favour of vaccination are making money out of it. On the other hand, doctors who oppose, or even question, vaccination, do not stand to gain anything but are, on the contrary, putting their careers at risk.

In case you decide to take the vaccine, ask the doctor to tell you the batch number of the vaccine. And keep the name of the doctor, the date and time, the batch number of the vaccine and the clinic address. Lawsuits against doctors, drug companies and the government usually fail because people do not have this information.

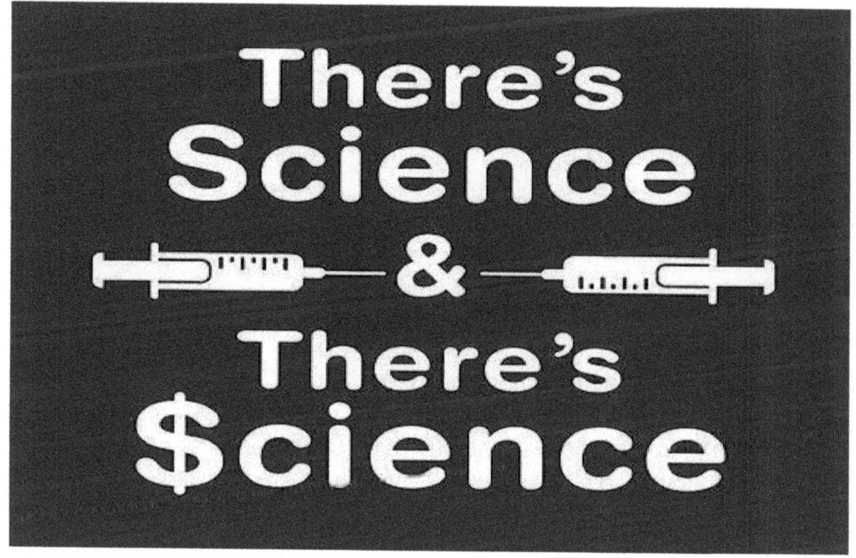

TERRAIN THEORY VS GERM THEORY

BANANA PEEL ANALOGY

If you do not throw a banana peel out into the garbage bin, but instead put it on your kitchen table. In a short period of time banana flies will start to feast on it. If you throw the banana peel into an effectively managed dustbin, the flies will disappear quickly.

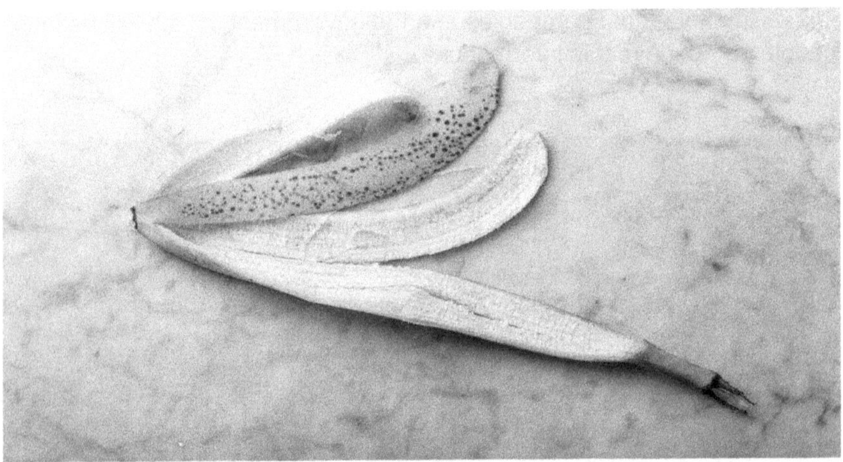

This means that the decomposing banana peel was the cause of the infestation of banana flies. If you remove the banana peel, they will not have anything to eat and will fly away to try to find another source of food or they will simply die. Of course, you could kill the flies, but without removing the banana peel you would only see new ones coming in. Same goes for micro-organisms, they are usually not the main cause of disease, but can give you a hard time if they get a chance to proliferate beyond your body's ability to cope with them. What conclusions can we draw from this example?

Well, keep your inner environment clean and in balance and the micro-organisms living in the body will work for you, not against you. They will not give you a hard time, because you do not interfere with nature. Many of them are actually necessary for you and will help you to maintain good health.[13] If we learn how to live according to the laws of nature, we do not have to fear the micro-organisms. The best prevention of disease is living a healthy lifestyle according to the laws of nature.

However, the real prevention of disease (living a healthy lifestyle) is unfortunately not taught at medical schools. The dogma of the germ theory of disease is pushed to all the medical students. It can sometimes be dangerous because they almost always see germs as the causative agents and treat the disease with antibiotics which does not help but often only makes things worse.

AQUARIUM ANALOGY

Imagine that you are a caretaker of an aquarium. You love and take care of the fish inside. Despite all your care, the water in the aquarium got polluted after a period of time. As a result, a fish starts falling sick.

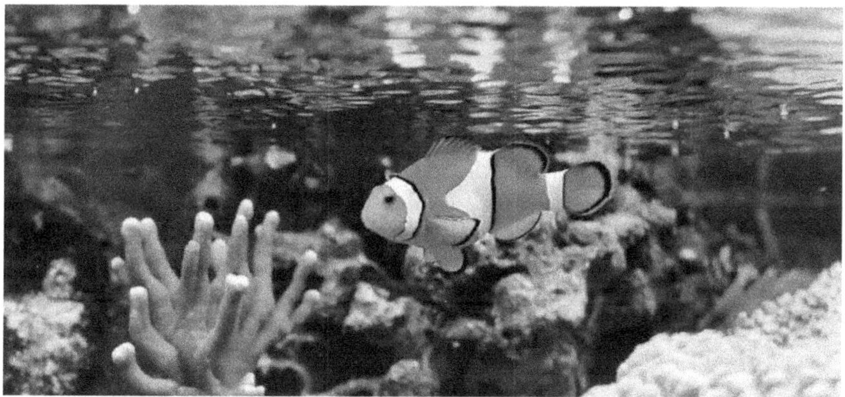

Now think yourself what you might have done if you or a member of your family fell sick. You would have visited the doctor! So, you decided to take the sick fish to a doctor. The doctor upon examining the fish gave some tablets and told that the fish must take it for a week and will be cured. You became happy when the fish started recovering. Since the water was still polluted, after some days the fish again fell sick. This time a little more serious. You did not want to take a chance. So, you decided to take the fish to the best hospital of the city. The doctor advised you to admit the fish in the hospital for a few days. Some injections and medication did the magic again. The fish recovered and got discharged from the hospital. You again dropped the fish into its house, i.e., aquarium. But again, after a few days the fish got seriously ill. This time the general physician referred him to a specialist and upon testing, the specialist doctor revealed that the fish is diabetic and must take metformin (diabetes pill) two times a day for the rest of its life and everything will be perfect. You trained the fish to follow the doctor's advice religiously. Despite all the best efforts from fish and you, after some time the fish fell ill again!

So, the question is what do you do now? Where is the problem? I know by now you must have already guessed the moral of the story. The problem was never in the fish! It was the polluted water! You simply must change the water. Even the best doctor of the world will not be able to cure the fish if it continues to live in the polluted water. Trying to cure the fish without finding the cause of the disease is like chasing a mirage. Every time it will appear that the cure is just nearby, but you will never be able to achieve it. In this process, you will drain your health and wealth.

Sometimes, to understand the solution you may not need the ultra-scientific approach towards the problem but just common sense, which most of the modern-day doctors lack. For example, diabetes type-2 is not a disease in which you require the knowledge of advanced microbiology to understand the problem. It is just a specific homeostatic condition of the body which can be understood and corrected with a change in diet and lifestyle.[14]

I have helped 100s of patients with type-2 diabetes reverse their diabetes by switching to a whole-food plant-based diet. Within few weeks of switching to this diet plan, their blood glucose readings start stabilizing and within a few months, they are able to maintain normal blood sugar readings without taking any medication like metformin. You can read about this process of natural healing in my book 'Advanced Nutrition Therapy: Goodbye Drugs and Diseases.'

Can we consume fruits in Type-2 Diabetes? Yes!

Study title: Fresh fruit consumption in relation to incident diabetes and diabetic vascular complications: A 7-y prospective study of 0.5 million Chinese adults; *PLoS Medicine, April 2017*

Description: In a large epidemiological study in over 500,000 Chinese adults, higher fresh fruit consumption was associated a 12% lower relative risk of developing diabetes and among diabetic individuals, 17% lower relative risk of dying from any cause and a 13%–28% lower risk of developing diabetes-related complications.[15] These findings suggested that a higher intake of fresh fruit is beneficial for prevention and treatment of diabetes.

Did your doctor tell you this? No!

MEDICAL SCIENCE OR MEDICAL CULTURE?

The following is an example of a common situation:

When someone gets injured by a rusted iron nail, the fear of tetanus prompts them to go for the tetanus vaccination. Here, we can consider two logical outcomes to accidentally stepping on a rusted nail:

1. The tetani bacteria was not present on the rusted nail and hence it did not enter your body. In this case, the tetanus vaccine is of no use.

2. Let's assume, the nail contained several tetani bacteria and through the injury, the tetani bacteria could invade the body.

Now post-injury, how would getting vaccinated against tetanus and adding some more fragments of tetani bacteria will help you to prevent the infection? This cannot be a science-based explanation. Rather the science says, "exposure to tetani toxin fragment by nerve terminals from an intramuscular depot (cuts and wounds) is an avid and rapid process and is not blocked by vaccination".[16]

Similarly post dog bite, going for rabies vaccination cannot be called as science rather a tradition followed under the influence of the profit minded pharmaceutical industry. Simply because, if the dog bite did not carry the "rabies virus" then the vaccine is not required anyway. If it did contain the "rabies virus" then the virus has already entered the body through the wound. If you take the vaccine after the dog bites you, then how would taking a weaker or inactive strand of the same virus prevent you from anything?

Tale of Medical Class (Allopathy)

Good morning, students! Today I welcome you all to the first day of medical college and you are going to learn about the medicine, and we are going to start with hypertension or high blood pressure. High blood pressure is quite common these days and we are going to talk about the medicines. There are several medicines, but we are going to talk about a medicine called diuretics which is considered very safe. The discomfort is very less and as soon as this medicine is given, the blood pressure becomes normal at once.

There are a few side effects of **Diuretics** such as erectile dysfunction, impotency, abnormal rhythms, palpitations, nausea, vomiting, headache, dizziness, joint pain, lethargy, tiredness, weakness but there is no need to worry. If a patient complains of erectile dysfunction, **Viagra** can be given but even after taking Viagra there are a few side effects like weakness, headache, dizziness, running nose, indigestion, etc. If a patient complains of headache after taking Viagra, he can be given **Paracetamol**. Even Paracetamol may lead to liver failure, constipation, or allergy, for which some other medicine can be provided.

The doctors have a solution for every problem in the form of medicine. For instance, for indigestion, **Zantac** can be recommended. Even after Zantac, a patient may complain of insomnia, diarrhea, nausea, or constipation, but again some medicine can be recommended. In the same way, for a person suffering from abnormal rhythm, **Pronestyl** can be given which may result in diarrhea or loss of appetite. If he complains of loss of appetite, he can be given **Imodium**. However, some side effects of Imodium are constipation, dizziness, abdominal pain, vomiting and nausea.

Diuretics	**Viagra**	**Paracetamol**	**Zantac**	**Pronestyl**
Impotency	Indigestion	Constipation	Constipation	Bitter taste
Joints pain	Runny nose	Allergy	Insomnia	Weakness
Weakness	Weakness	Liver failure	Weakness	Headache
Headache	Headache	Jaundice	Headache	Nausea
Nausea	Backache	Nausea	Nausea	Dizziness
Palpitations	Redness	Diarrhea	Diarrhea	Diarrhea
Dizziness	Dizziness	Stomach pain	Dizziness	Appetite loss

So, in this way, the list of medicines keeps increasing and at the end of the day, the patient himself forgets the problem for which he had initially consulted the doctor. He just remembers the medicines to be taken in the morning, afternoon, and night. He starts taking medicines as food and feels that he is protected because of these medicines. This is enough for you to understand that the patient is now going to drown in a whirlpool of problems.

As reported in 2015, in the Huffington Post, "Those aged 65 to 69 take an average of 15 prescriptions per year, while those from 80 to 84 take an average of 18, according to the American Association of Consultant Pharmacists."[17] The report says that on average, 45-year-olds take 4 prescription drugs every day! This is called polypharmacy and it is killing thousands of Americans annually. According to FDA statistics 1.3 million people are injured annually due to medication error.[18]

The Vicious Cycle of Medications: Chronic Diseases create demand for other Medications and Surgeries

The evidence of a connection between vaccines and autoimmune diseases is strong and growing. So, how are the vaccine makers responding to that? They are making new vaccines against autoimmune diseases![19] This exemplifies the mindset of pharmaceutical companies. First treat symptoms with a medication that creates other symptoms, then treat those symptoms with another medication that creates other symptoms. And around and around you go!

If vaccines are at least in part responsible for the rising prevalence of autoimmune diseases, how is creating more vaccines to treat the autoimmune diseases going to solve the problem? They try to fix the problem with the same approach that caused the problem in the first place. Vaccines like other medications, create a huge demand for other medications and medical care at an extremely high cost! Rather than accepting responsibility for the contribution of a product to an epidemic of autoimmune diseases, they see it as opportunity for an additional market share.

INGREDIENTS OF VACCINES: IT WILL SHOCK YOU

Some of the things that you will see in vaccine ingredients list are:

Aluminum and thimerosal (mercury) which are highly neurotoxic heavy metals; **formaldehyde** (formalin) is a proven carcinogen; **monosodium glutamate** (MSG) is a neuroexcitatory chemical; **fetal cow serum** (made by killing pregnant cows); **2-phenoxyethanol** that the FDA has associated with depression of the central nervous system; cell cultures from aborted babies; **monkey kidney cells** (VERO cells); **antibiotics** like neomycin, neomycin sulfate, kanamycin, streptomycin, tetracycline and gentamicin sulfate; **polysorbate-80** (tween 80) and **polysorbate-20**; **nonylphenol ethoxylate**; **acetone**; unique animal derived **retroviruses** that have been found in human tumors and tissues; **human serum albumin**; human and **animal DNA** (even DNA fragments from the **aborted human fetuses** mentioned above); **serum proteins of human, cow, chicken and pig**; **glutaraldehyde** which is a strong biocide disinfectant for industrial purposes; **squalene**; **cetyltrimethylammonium bromide**; **β-propiolactone** plus many other chemicals with names that are difficult, if not impossible to pronounce. Do you really think that any of these will contribute to your health in any form?

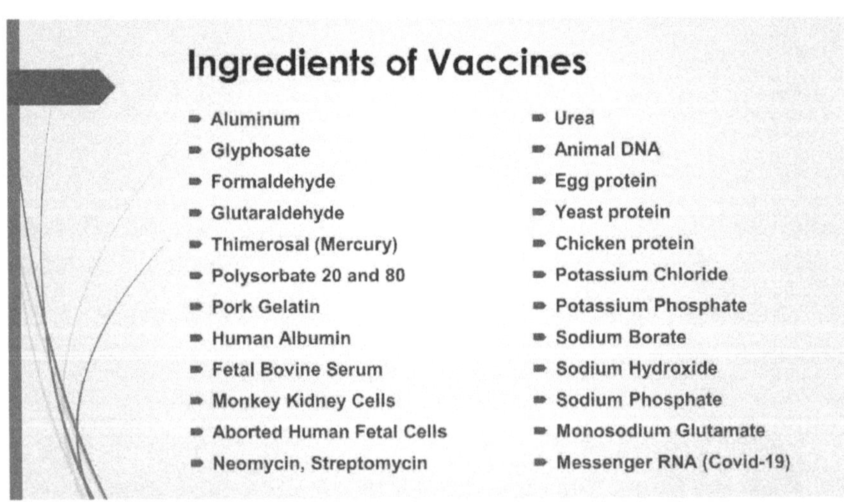

On the next pages you can read specific ingredients for specific vaccines.[20] You will get shocked to see that what you considered as preventive treatments are extremely toxic and poisonous to inject in your blood.

Vaccine Excipient Table

Vaccine (Trade Name)	Package Insert Date	Contains[a]
Adenovirus	10/2019	monosodium glutamate, sucrose, D-mannose, D-fructose, dextrose, human serum albumin, potassium phosphate, plasdone C, anhydrous lactose, microcrystalline cellulose, polacrilin potassium, magnesium stearate, cellulose acetate phthalate, alcohol, acetone, castor oil, FD&C Yellow #6 aluminum lake dye
Anthrax (Biothrax)	11/2015	aluminum hydroxide, sodium chloride, benzethonium chloride, formaldehyde
BCG (Tice)	02/2009	glycerin, asparagine, citric acid, potassium phosphate, magnesium sulfate, iron ammonium citrate, lactose
Cholera (Vaxchora)	06/2016	ascorbic acid, hydrolyzed casein, sodium chloride, sucrose, dried lactose, sodium bicarbonate, sodium carbonate
Dengue (Dengvaxia)	06/2019	sodium chloride, essential amino acids (including L-phenylalanine), non-essential amino acids, L-arginine hydrochloride, sucrose, D-trehalose dihydrate, D-sorbitol, trometamol, urea
DT (Sanofi)	06/2018	aluminum phosphate, isotonic sodium chloride, formaldehyde
DTaP (Daptacel)	01/2021[b]	aluminum phosphate, formaldehyde, glutaraldehyde, 2-phenoxyethanol
DTaP (Infanrix)	01/2021[b]	formaldehyde, aluminum hydroxide, sodium chloride, polysorbate 80 (Tween 80)
DTaP-IPV (Kinrix)	01/2021[b]	formaldehyde, aluminum hydroxide, sodium chloride, polysorbate 80 (Tween 80), neomycin sulfate, polymyxin B
DTaP-IPV (Quadracel)	02/2021	formaldehyde, aluminum phosphate, 2-phenoxyethanol, polysorbate 80, glutaraldehyde, neomycin, polymyxin B sulfate, bovine serum albumin
DTaP-HepB-IPV (Pediarix)	01/2021[b]	formaldehyde, aluminum hydroxide, aluminum phosphate, sodium chloride, polysorbate 80 (Tween 80), neomycin sulfate, polymyxin B, yeast protein
DTaP-IPV/Hib (Pentacel)	12/2019	aluminum phosphate, polysorbate 80, sucrose, formaldehyde, glutaraldehyde, bovine serum albumin, 2-phenoxyethanol, neomycin, polymyxin B sulfate
DTaP-IPV-Hib-HepB (Vaxelis)	10/2020	polysorbate 80, formaldehyde, glutaraldehyde, bovine serum albumin, neomycin, streptomycin sulfate, polymyxin B sulfate, ammonium thiocyanate, yeast protein, aluminum
Ebola Zaire (ERVEBO)	01/2021[b]	Tromethamine, rice-derived recombinant human serum albumin, host cell DNA, benzonase, rice protein
Hib (ActHIB)	05/2019	sodium chloride, formaldehyde, sucrose
Hib (Hiberix)	04/2018	formaldehyde, sodium chloride, lactose
Hib (PedvaxHIB)	01/2021[b]	amorphous aluminum hydroxyphosphate sulfate, sodium chloride
Hep A (Havrix)	01/2021[b]	MRC-5 cellular proteins, formalin, aluminum hydroxide, amino acid supplement, phosphate-buffered saline solution, polysorbate 20, neomycin sulfate, aminoglycoside antibiotic
Hep A (Vaqta)	01/2021[b]	amorphous aluminum hydroxyphosphate sulfate, non-viral protein, DNA, bovine albumin, formaldehyde, neomycin, sodium borate, sodium chloride, other process chemical residuals
Hep B (Engerix-B)	01/2021[b]	aluminum hydroxide, yeast protein, sodium chloride, disodium phosphate dihydrate, sodium dihydrogen phosphate dihydrate
Hep B (Recombivax)	12/2018	formaldehyde, potassium aluminum sulfate, amorphous aluminum hydroxyphosphate sulfate, yeast protein
Hep B (Heplisav-B)	05/2020	yeast protein, yeast DNA, deoxycholate, phosphorothioate linked oligodeoxynucleotide, sodium phosphate, dibasic dodecahydrate, sodium chloride, monobasic dehydrate, polysorbate 80
Hep A/Hep B (Twinrix)	01/2021[b]	MRC-5 cellular proteins, formalin, aluminum phosphate, aluminum hydroxide, amino acids, sodium chloride, phosphate buffer, polysorbate 20, neomycin sulfate, yeast protein
HPV (Gardasil 9)	08/2020	amorphous aluminum hydroxyphosphate sulfate, sodium chloride, L-histidine, polysorbate 80, sodium borate, yeast protein

Vaccine (Trade Name)	Package Insert Date	Contains[a]
Influenza (Afluria) Quadrivalent[c]	03/2021	sodium chloride, monobasic sodium phosphate, dibasic sodium phosphate, monobasic potassium phosphate, potassium chloride, calcium chloride, sodium taurodeoxycholate, ovalbumin, sucrose, neomycin sulfate, polymyxin B, beta-propiolactone, hydrocortisone, thimerosal (multi-dose vials)
Influenza (Fluad) Quadrivalent[c]	03/2021	squalene, polysorbate 80, sorbitan trioleate, sodium citrate dihydrate, citric acid monohydrate, neomycin, kanamycin, hydrocortisone, egg protein, formaldehyde
Influenza (Fluarix) Quadrivalent[c]	2021	octoxynol-10 (TRITON X-100), α-tocopheryl hydrogen succinate, polysorbate 80 (Tween 80), hydrocortisone, gentamicin sulfate, ovalbumin, formaldehyde, sodium deoxycholate, sodium phosphate-buffered isotonic sodium chloride
Influenza (Flublok) Quadrivalent[c]	03/2021	sodium chloride, monobasic sodium phosphate, dibasic sodium phosphate, polysorbate 20 (Tween 20), baculovirus and *Spodoptera frugiperda* cell proteins, baculovirus and cellular DNA, Triton X-100
Influenza (Flucelvax) Quadrivalent[c]	10/2021[b]	Madin Darby Canine Kidney (MDCK) cell protein, phosphate buffered saline, protein other than HA, MDCK cell DNA, polysorbate 80, cetyltrimethlyammonium bromide, and β-propiolactone, thimerosal (multi-dose vials)
Influenza (Flulaval) Quadrivalent[c]	2021	ovalbumin, formaldehyde, sodium deoxycholate, α-tocopheryl hydrogen succinate, polysorbate 80, phosphate-buffered saline solution
Influenza (Fluzone) Quadrivalent[c]	2021	formaldehyde, egg protein, octylphenol ethoxylate (Triton X-100), sodium phosphate-buffered isotonic sodium chloride solution, thimerosal (multi-dose vials)
Influenza (Fluzone) High Dose[c]	07/2021	egg protein, octylphenol ethoxylate (Triton X-100), sodium phosphate-buffered isotonic sodium chloride solution, formaldehyde
Influenza (FluMist) Quadrivalent[c]	08/2021	monosodium glutamate, hydrolyzed porcine gelatin, arginine, sucrose, dibasic potassium phosphate, monobasic potassium phosphate, ovalbumin, gentamicin sulfate, ethylenediaminetetraacetic acid (EDTA)
IPV (Ipol)	01/2021[b]	calf bovine serum albumin, 2-phenoxyethanol, formaldehyde, neomycin, streptomycin, polymyxin B, M-199 medium
Japanese Encephalitis (Ixiaro)	09/2018	aluminum hydroxide, protamine sulfate, formaldehyde, bovine serum albumin, host cell DNA, sodium metabisulphite, host cell protein
MenACWY (Menactra)	04/2018	sodium phosphate buffered isotonic sodium chloride solution, formaldehyde, diphtheria toxoid protein carrier
MenACWY (MenQuadfi)	01/2021[b]	sodium chloride, sodium acetate, formaldehyde
MenACWY (Menveo)	07/2020	formaldehyde, CRM_{197} protein
MenB (Bexsero)	01/2021[b]	aluminum hydroxide, sodium chloride, histidine, sucrose, kanamycin
MenB (Trumenba)	2018	polysorbate 80, aluminum phosphate, histidine buffered saline
MMR (MMR-II)	12/2020	sorbitol, sucrose, hydrolyzed gelatin, recombinant human albumin, neomycin, fetal bovine serum, WI-38 human diploid lung fibroblasts
MMRV (ProQuad) (Frozen: Recombinant Albumin)	01/2021[b]	MRC-5 cells including DNA and protein, sucrose, hydrolyzed gelatin, sodium chloride, sorbitol, monosodium L-glutamate, sodium phosphate dibasic, recombinant human albumin, sodium bicarbonate, potassium phosphate monobasic, potassium chloride, potassium phosphate dibasic, neomycin, bovine calf serum, other buffer and media ingredients
PCV13 (Prevnar 13)	08/2017	CRM_{197} carrier protein, polysorbate 80, succinate buffer, aluminum phosphate
PPSV-23 (Pneumovax)	09/2020	isotonic saline solution, phenol
Rabies (Imovax)	10/2019	human albumin, neomycin sulfate, phenol red, beta-propiolactone
Rabies (RabAvert)	2018	chicken protein, polygeline (processed bovine gelatin), human serum albumin, potassium glutamate, sodium EDTA, ovalbumin, neomycin, chlortetracycline, amphotericin B
Rotavirus (RotaTeq)	01/2021[b]	sucrose, sodium citrate, sodium phosphate monobasic monohydrate, sodium hydroxide, polysorbate 80, cell culture media, fetal bovine serum

Vaccine (Trade Name)	Package Insert Date	Contains[a]
Rotavirus (Rotarix)	01/2021[b]	dextran, Dulbecco's Modified Eagle Medium (sodium chloride, potassium chloride, magnesium sulfate, ferric (III) nitrate, sodium phosphate, sodium pyruvate, D-glucose, concentrated vitamin solution, L-cystine, L-tyrosine, amino acids, L-glutamine, calcium chloride, sodium hydrogenocarbonate, and phenol red), sorbitol, sucrose, calcium carbonate, sterile water, xanthan [Porcine circovirus type 1 (PCV1) is present in Rotarix. PCV-1 is not known to cause disease in humans.]
Smallpox (Vaccinia) (ACAM2000)	03/2018	HEPES, 2% human serum albumin, 0.5 - 0.7% sodium chloride USP, 5% Mannitol USP, neomycin, polymyxin B, 50% Glycerin USP, 0.25% phenol USP
Td (Tenivac)	11/2019	aluminum phosphate, formaldehyde, sodium chloride
Td (TDVAX)	09/2018	aluminum phosphate, formaldehyde, thimerosal
Tdap (Adacel)	12/2020	aluminum phosphate, formaldehyde, 2-phenoxyethanol, glutaraldehyde
Tdap (Boostrix)	09/2020	formaldehyde, aluminum hydroxide, sodium chloride, polysorbate 80
Typhoid (Typhim Vi)	03/2020	formaldehyde, phenol, polydimethylsiloxane, disodium phosphate, monosodium phosphate, sodium chloride
Typhoid (Vivotif Ty21a)	9/2013	sucrose, ascorbic acid, amino acids, lactose, magnesium stearate, gelatin
Varicella (Varivax) Frozen	01/2021[b]	sucrose, hydrolyzed gelatin, sodium chloride, monosodium L-glutamate, sodium phosphate dibasic, potassium phosphate monobasic, potassium chloride, MRC-5 human diploid cells including DNA & protein, sodium phosphate monobasic, EDTA, neomycin, fetal bovine serum
Yellow Fever (YF-Vax)	2/2019	sorbitol, gelatin, sodium chloride
Zoster (Shingles) (Shingrix)	01/2021[b]	sucrose, sodium chloride, dioleoyl phosphatidylcholine (DOPC), 3-*O*-desacl-4'monophosphoryl lipid A (MPL), QS-21 (a saponin purified from plant extract *Quillaja saponaria* Molina), potassium dihydrogen phosphate, cholesterol, sodium dihydrogen phosphate dihydrate, disodium phosphate anhydrous, dipotassium phosphate, polysorbate 80, host cell protein and DNA

Update: As of January 2019, the CDC has changed the way they are reporting the vaccine ingredients on their vaccine excipient and media table. They have removed the word media from the title and have added the following statement – "Note: Substances used in the manufacture of a vaccine but not listed as contained in the final product (e.g., culture media) can be found in each product insert but are not shown on this table." This is very problematic because it appears as though they do not want to be fully forthcoming with the public who want to know what exactly is in the vaccines. It is possible for an individual to go to each vaccine's product insert online and find the ingredient section and read it there, but that is very tedious and time consuming.

It also looks as though they have removed the WI-38 Human Diploid Lung Fibroblasts Cell line that the virus for the Rubella portion of the MMR and MMRV vaccines are cultured in. Those human lung fibroblasts came from an aborted baby in 1962. In fact, the baby used was the 32nd aborted baby they used before settling on these cells. The cells containing that baby's own DNA have been used since that time. This is problematic on many levels, including moral, ethical, religious, and potential for causing health problems in humans including the possibility that this DNA could contaminate the DNA of the person getting the vaccines.

Direct access to the package inserts of all vaccines containing all the ingredients can be found here: http://www.immunize.org/fda/

✦ THIMEROSAL (MERCURY):

Robert F. Kennedy's organization World Mercury Project released a 248-page eBook titled Peer-Reviewed, Published Research on the Adverse Effects of Mercury. It is a compilation of over 240 studies detailing the toxicology and health damaging effects of mercury.[21]

A study published in the Journal of Toxicological and Environmental Chemistry found that Thimerosal damaged brain cells even in very small quantities.[22]

From the study: "Routine administering of Thimerosal-containing biologics/childhood vaccines have become significant sources of Hg exposure for some fetuses/infants." "Thimerosal at low nanomolar concentrations induced significant cellular toxicity in human neuronal and fetal cells. Thimerosal-induced cytoxicity (cell toxicity) is similar to that observed in AD (Alzheimer's Disease), pathophysiologic studies. Thimerosal was found to be significantly more toxic than the other metal compounds examined."

Another study published in International Journal of Clinical Chemistry concluded that "thimerosal is a poison at minute levels with a plethora of deleterious consequences even at the levels currently administered in vaccines."[23]

✦ ALUMINUM:

Environmental influences including aluminum vaccine adjuvants are triggers for the development of autism.[24] A study published in Journal of Environment International looked at the full spectrum of environmental factors that can be contributing factors in the genesis of autism. But the last sentence seems to put an exclamation point on the aluminum from adjuvants.

From the Abstract: "In developed countries, it is now reported that 1%-1.5% of children have ASD, and in the US 2015 CDC reports that approximately one in 45 children suffer from ASD." "A comprehensive literature search has implicated several environmental factors associated with the development of ASD. These include pesticides, phthalates, polychlorinated biphenyls, solvents, air pollutants, fragrances, glyphosate, and heavy metals, especially aluminum used in vaccines as adjuvant."

✚ 2-PHENOXYETHANOL:

In 2008, the FDA has warned consumers against using nipple creams for breastfeeding mothers because the phenoxyethanol in it "can depress the central nervous system and may cause vomiting and diarrhea, which can lead to dehydration in infants."[25] So, something that can potentially depress the central nervous system is directly being injected in the bloodstream of children through vaccines. Why?

✚ POLYSORBATE-80:

An article from the Annals of Allergy, Asthma & Immunology showed that Polysorbate 80 which is one of the common ingredients in vaccines can cause anaphylactic reactions. According to the article, "Polysorbate 80 was identified as the causative agent for the anaphylactoid reaction of nonimmunologic origin." The article concluded that, "Polysorbate 80 is a ubiquitously used solubilizing agent that can cause severe nonimmunologic anaphylactoid reactions."[26]

✚ FORMALDEHYDE (FORMALIN):

Formaldehyde is toxic and known to cause cancer. The International Agency for Research on Cancer (IARC) classifies formaldehyde as a human carcinogen. It is proven to cause nasopharyngeal cancer, sinonasal cancer, and myeloid leukemia.[27]

✚ BETA-PROPIOLACTONE:

According to Wikipedia, Beta-Propiolactone is made industrially by the reaction of formaldehyde and ethenone. It is an excellent sterilizing and sporicidal agent, but its carcinogenicity precludes that use. β-Propiolactone is reasonably anticipated to be a human carcinogen.[28] [29]

Beta-Propiolactone is classified as a potential human carcinogen on the Occupational Safety and Health Guideline found on the CDC's website. In its summary of toxicology under the heading 'effects on animals', it is mentioned that "In rats, acute oral administration, or intraperitoneal injection of beta-propiolactone caused muscular spasms, respiratory difficulty, convulsions, and death. Acute intravenous injection caused kidney tubule and liver damage. Subcutaneous injection of β-propiolactone in rats and mice produced cancer at the sites of administration. Single intraperitoneal injections in suckling mice produced tumors and liver cancer."[30]

According to New Jersey Department of Health and Senior Services, "Beta-Propiolactone should be handled as a carcinogen with extreme caution. It is a corrosive chemical which can severely irritate and burn the eyes with possible permanent damage. It may be carcinogenic in humans since it has been shown to cause skin and stomach cancers in animals."[31]

GLUTARALDEHYDE:

It is an organic compound that is used to disinfect medical and dental equipment. In vaccines, it is used as a chemical preservative. There have been several studies done on Glutaraldehyde and it has been found that exposure to it can cause asthma, allergic reactions, induced respiratory issues, diarrhea, etc.[32]

PHENOL (CARBOLIC ACID):

Phenol is a known mutagen, (meaning it causes cells to mutate), a teratogen (meaning causes birth defects), and fetotoxic (or toxic to the fetus). According to the Material Safety Data Sheet (MSDS), "Phenol may be toxic to kidneys, liver, central nervous system (CNS). Repeated or prolonged exposure to the substance can produce target organs damage".[33] "Phenol is also considered to be an extremely hazardous substance." according to the EPA cited in a CDC document.[34] Yet, with all that evidence on phenol, the CDC recommends vaccines containing phenol for pregnant women.

ENDOCRINE DISRUPTING CHEMICALS (NPEs and OPEs):

Nonylphenol Ethoxylate (NPEs): NPEs are non-ionic surfactants that are used in a wide variety of industrial applications and consumer products. Many of these, such as laundry detergents, are "down-the-drain" applications. NPEs, though less toxic and persistent than NP, are also highly toxic to aquatic organisms, and, in the environment, degrade into NP. NP has also been shown to exhibit estrogenic properties in in vitro and in vivo assays. Nonylphenol is also neurotoxic. Nonylphenol has been reported to have deleterious effects on central nervous system (CNS) other than reproductive and immune systems including disrupting neuroendocrine homeostasis, altering cognitive function, and neurotoxicity of tissues, etc.[35]

Octylphenol ethoxylate (OPEs) and Octoxynol-10: It is also known as Triton X-100. It is closely related to Nonylphenol Ethoxylate. OPEs function as a detergent and are widely used in cleaning agents. They are also added to paints, coatings, treatments for textiles and chemicals used in paper manufacture. According to Wikipedia, Triton X-100 is widely used to lyse cells to extract protein or organelles, or to permeabilize the membranes of living cells.

CETYLTRIMETHYLAMMONIUM BROMIDE:

According to the Material Safety Data Sheet, "there is some evidence that human exposure to the material may result in developmental toxicity."[36] It is considered a hazardous substance according to Occupational Safety and Health Administration.

KANAMYCIN, NEOMYCIN AND GENTAMICIN SULFATE:

These antibiotics are contraindicated (not recommended), for pregnant women or nursing mothers. However, these are found in several flu vaccines and the CDC recommends the flu vaccine for all pregnant women. These antibiotics are in the same family of antibiotics called aminoglycosides. According to the warning label, "Aminoglycosides can cause fetal harm when administered to pregnant women. Aminoglycoside antibiotics cross the placenta and there have been several reports of total, irreversible, bilateral congenital deafness in children whose mothers' received streptomycin during pregnancy." The warning label of these antibiotics state "This medication is not recommended for use during pregnancy."[37]

SQUALENE:

Squalene is a colorless poly-unsaturated hydrocarbon liquid that's found naturally in many animals and plants, including human sebum. Essentially, it's one of the many natural lipids our body produces to lubricate and protect our skin. Squalene itself is not dangerous, but when it is injected, the body's immune system over-reacts and produces antibodies that attack all the other squalene in the body, including in places where it can be beneficial like your nervous system and other organs and tissues. In a study published in the American Journal of Pathology, they injected squalene into arthritis prone rats that caused them to develop rheumatoid arthritis.[38]

SODIUM BORATE (BORAX):

Sodium Borate is a common ingredient found in rat poison, pesticides, and various commercial applications such as flame retardants, enamel glazes, and laundry detergent. According to one source, the U.S. National Library of Medicine states in an article that boric acid is no longer commonly used in medical preparations as this substance was used to disinfect and treat wounds and the individuals who received such treatment got sick, and some died.[39]

"Because of reproductive and developmental toxicity concerns, borax was added to the European Union's (EU) Substance of Very High Concern (SVHC) candidate list in December 2010. The SVHC candidate list is part of the EU Regulations on the Registration, Evaluation, Authorization and Restriction of Chemicals 2006, and the addition was based on the revised classification of borax as toxic for reproduction category 1B under the Classification, Labeling and Packaging Regulations. Substances and mixtures imported into the EU which contain borax are now required to be labeled with the warnings 'May damage fertility' and 'May damage the unborn child'."[40]

VERO CELLS:

These are cell lines from the African Green Monkey kidney cultures. Vaccines such as the Smallpox vaccine using live Smallpox virus grown in the VERO cells have a laundry list of serious potential side effects. The following is from the Smallpox Vaccine package insert and can be found on the FDA's website. Under the warning it can be read that "Suspected cases of myocarditis and/or pericarditis have been observed in healthy adult primary vaccinees."[41]

"Encephalitis, encephalomyelitis, encephalopathy, progressive vaccinia, generalized vaccinia, severe vaccinial skin infections, erythema multiforme major (including stevens-johnson syndrome), eczema vaccinatum resulting in permanent sequelae or death, ocular complications, blindness, and fetal death have occurred following either primary vaccination or revaccination with live vaccinia virus smallpox vaccines." "The risk for experiencing serious vaccination complications must be weighed against the risks for experiencing a potentially fatal smallpox infection."

Another 2018 study also verifies this danger of myocarditis following smallpox vaccination. The study published in the British Medical Journal Case Reports states that "vaccines are not without risk; reactions can range from injection site reactions to life-threatening anaphylaxis. Among the more serious vaccine-related sequela is myocarditis. Although myocarditis has been reported following many different vaccines, the smallpox vaccine has the strongest association."[42]

⍿ UNDISCLOSED INGREDIENTS:

An article published in the International Journal of Vaccines and Vaccination reveals a shocking conglomeration of non-biocompatible particulates and foreign bodies in randomly selected batches of 43 different human vaccines and one veterinary vaccine.[43]

The introduction of the article also has much to say about the known side effects of vaccines. "Side effects have always been reported but in the latest years it seems that they have increased in number and seriousness, particularly in children as the American Academy of pediatrics reports. "For instance, the diphtheria-tetanus-pertussis (DTaP) vaccine was linked to cases of sudden infant death syndrome (SIDS); (MMR) measles-mumps-rubella vaccine with autism; multiple immunizations with immune disorders; hepatitis B vaccines with multiple sclerosis, etc."

The study concludes that, "All samples checked vaccines contain non biocompatible and bio-persistent foreign bodies which are not declared by the Producers, against which the body reacts in any case."

They also found aluminum in some vaccines that do not list in in the ingredients list. Also discovered was lead, stainless steel, tungsten, silicon, gold, silver, nickel, iron, chromium, copper, zirconium, Hafnium, Strontium, Antimony, Platinum, Bismuth, Cerium, and aggregates of combinations of these metals and biological compounds the researchers called nano-bio-interactions. This means that all the human vaccines contain unintended particulates and aggregates of metals and foreign matter, most likely from the manufacturing process.

MORAL, ETHICAL, AND RELIGIOUS CONCERNS AROUND VACCINES (USE OF ABORTED BABIES)

Aborted fetal cells are also used in the development and/or production of vaccines. This raises serious religious, personal, ethical, and moral issues. Abortion is a contentious issue because unborn babies are killed. The injection of DNA from aborted fetal cell lines into a person's body in unconscionable to many based on their beliefs. Most of the people have no idea that they were allowing these DNA particulates from aborted babies to be injected into their bodies. There is often no true informed consent with vaccines. Inadequate vaccine related information is provided to most people which does not allow them to make a well evaluated decision. People should be told everything about the ingredients. The following is a brief description of the aborted fetal cells used in vaccines:

- The **WI-38** cell line was developed by Dr. Leonard Hayflick in 1962, by taking lung tissue from an aborted baby. The WI comes from Wistar Institute and the 38 is the number of aborted babies used until they found the "perfect" cell line for their purposes.

- The **MRC-5** cell line was developed for the Medical Research Council in England by J.P. Jacobs in 1966 from lung tissue of an aborted baby. These are vaccines that contain human DNA and aborted fetal tissue from these cell lines: Adenovirus, DTaP, hepatitis A, hepatitis B, MMR, MMRV, rabies, varicella (Chickenpox) and zoster (Shingles).

- The **HEK-293** is used for research (and vaccines). This cell line originated from a legally aborted fetus in the Netherlands in 1973. The tissue came from the baby's kidneys, hence Human Embryonic Kidney (HEK). The lab culturing the cells was Alex van der Eb's laboratory. Frank Graham was the scientist running the experiments refining the cell culture process. The 293 was incorporated in the name because it was produced from his 293rd experiment. Current vaccines that contain DNA from this cell line are for Covid-19, Cystic Fibrosis, Ebola, Heart (Abciximab-Repro), Hemophilia, Infection prevention (G-CSF).

- The **PER.C6** cell line is a line that is not only being used in vaccine production, but also in many other medicines. It was developed in 1995. The PER.C6 cell line is derived from human embryonic retinal cells, originally from the retinal tissue of an 18-week-old fetus aborted in 1985 and further developed and prepared as cell line by transfection with defined E1 region of the adenovirus type 5 followed by selection for transfectants with an immortal phenotype.[44]

- The **walvax-2** cell line is the most recent development of human fetal cell lines from an aborted baby. In an article in Journal of Human Vaccines and Immunotherapeutics, it is discussed that the walvax-2 cell line will eventually take the place of the MRC-5 and the WI-38 lines as they lose the ability to self-replicate.[45]

  The Ethics of the Walvax-2 Cell Strain[46]: There were 9 aborted fetuses "competing" for the one that produced the best cell line (walvax-2) to make vaccines from. The cells eventually used, came from lung tissue of a 3-month-old female aborted baby in China. The method they used to deliver the fetus was the "water bag" method, which was done to deliver the baby intact, to provide the freshest and most viable tissue samples possible. The tissues from the freshly aborted fetuses were immediately sent to the laboratory for the preparation of the cells.

The question of whether a fetus is a human life or not has created polarizing battles in our nation. To take it to the next level, this methodology brings into question a whole other moral and ethical dilemma as to whether a fetus should be terminated (killed) inside or outside the womb. Does it suffer more if killed before being delivered alive or not. I am sure many people reading this book have never thought this way. To witness and experience the pain, suffering and aftermath of the baby that you are killing, without conscious or self-remorse is beyond me.

Other aborted fetal cell lines are also used for vaccines and medical/scientific purposes. Numerous other cell strains have been made as back-ups for the current strains, and for research. Two of the most known stains are:

- **MRC-9** (Medical Research Council cell strain 9) was derived from the lungs of a female fetus aborted in 1974 and developed by Jacobs and colleagues for research and as a back-up for vaccine manufacture.

- **IMR-90** (Institute for Medical Research cell strain 90) was derived from the lungs of a sixteen-week-old female fetus aborted in July 1975. IMR-90 is designated for "research and related activities."

This PDF lists all vaccines that have DNA from aborted fetuses:
https://cogforlife.org/wp-content/uploads/vaccineListOrigFormat.pdf

If you think that vaccines do not contain aborted fetal cells then read the article titled, Development of Vaccines from Aborted Babies by Jessica Farnsworth, M.D., May 2011. This paper discusses the history of using aborted babies to produce the cell lines that are still used in many of the vaccines today.[49]

DEOXYRIBONUCLEIC ACID (DNA)

DNA is harvested from the aborted fetuses cell lines. It is used as adjuvant in vaccines. In vaccines, 100,000,000 bits and strands of human DNA are allowed per dose according to FDA. We have human DNA, human cell lines from aborted infants, and protein from human blood in 23 of our vaccines.

When we need a blood transfusion, or a blood donation of some kind, what is absolutely required? A match, correct? For example, if a person with type O blood receives type A+ blood, the outcome is fatal. There are rules of science that cannot be crossed regarding DNA and blood. It is imperative to be evaluated when receiving any type of tissue or blood to ensure that a fatal blood or tissue type is not put into your body. So, may I ask: How many of you or your children were given a blood test before receiving vaccinations? We all know the answer to that. It does not happen. The outcome to mixing without matching human blood and tissue with other humans can be virtually disastrous.

In addition to the obvious reason for a person of faith to decline having that DNA injected into their body, there is also concern among many scientists that these DNA fragments can combine with the recipient's DNA in a process called homologous recombination and that the resultant inflammatory reaction may lead to autoimmune responses and other downstream effects of the alteration of the recipients DNA including triggering inflammation in the brain leading to regressive autism in genetically susceptible children. There is such evidence showing that when human DNA was incorporated into vaccines, there was a significant uptick in the rate of autism. A 2014 article published in the Journal of Public Health and Epidemiology produces convincing evidence of the effects of human fetal cell lines on the "change point" where the incidence of autism rose sharply in the late 1980s.[47]

MMR Vaccine is Associated with Autism Spectrum Disorder (This Vaccine is Produced in Aborted Fetal Cell Lines)

A Natural Experiment: Rate of Autism dropped as MMR vaccine compliance rates dropped and as MMR vaccine compliance rates increased again, so did rates of autism. It shows a positive relation with MMR vaccine uptake and autism rates.

Study title: Epidemiologic and Molecular Relationship Between Vaccine Manufacture and Autism Spectrum Disorder Prevalence[48]; *Issues in Law and Medicine, 2015*

Description: This article reveals that when Dr. Andrew Wakefield identified gastrointestinal pathological changes in children that reacted to the MMR vaccine and many parents pulled back from having their children vaccinated with MMR, there was a corresponding temporary drop in rates of diagnosed Autism Spectrum Disorder for those children that fell within those birth years. And as interestingly, when the rates of MMR compliance once again recovered, the rates of Autism increased proportionately. The article also reveals the contribution to and risk of foreign human fetal DNA contamination into DNA of vaccine recipients, the relationship with Autism and the associated health risks involved.

From the article: "The average MMR coverage for the three countries fell below 90% after Dr. Wakefield's infamous 1998 publication but started to recover slowly after 2001 until reaching over 90% coverage again by 2004. During the same time period, the average autism spectrum disorder prevalence in the United Kingdom, Norway and Sweden dropped substantially after birth year 1998 and gradually increased again after birth year 2000."

My opinion of vaccines made with Aborted Fetal Cells:

I am a Sikh, and as such I cannot use a product that was developed from the abortion industry, even if it means great inconvenience or even danger for my family. The evil performed when these babies were killed decades ago is sufficient to make these tainted vaccines morally unacceptable. Also, I am convinced that all the current vaccines are useless for mankind and carry potential life-threatening dangers. Millions of babies are killed by abortion around the world each year. How can we say that the pharmaceutical industry is not contributing to this evil? And how can we participate in this evil?

As a person with extraordinarily strong Sikh faith and conviction, I feel that the human DNA from aborted fetal cell lines used in the MMR and many of the other vaccines, violate the sanctity of human life.

"*In the first watch of the night, O my merchant friend, you were cast into the womb, by the Lord's Command.*" (Sri Guru Granth Sahib Ji, Angg 74)

As stated in the holy scripture of Sri Guru Granth Sahib Ji, human life begins at conception and the science is also incontrovertible on that. Abortion is clearly the termination of a human life. As such, I am strongly opposed to abortion and the sale of aborted babies or their body parts. This would most certainly be an abomination in God's eyes. And horrifically, in many cases these babies were intentionally delivered alive before being killed for their tissues. And for each baby used, there were dozens of ones that were not used as they did not make a good match for what the "scientists" were looking for.

"*This body is the Temple of the Lord, in which the jewel of spiritual wisdom is revealed.*" (Sri Guru Granth Sahib Ji, Angg 1346)

As stated in the holy scripture of Sri Guru Granth Sahib Ji, human body is the Temple of God. Vaccines contain many other toxic ingredients in addition to the residual human DNA from the aborted babies that are in direct conflict with the way a Sikh of Guru Granth Sahib Ji would honor the human body.

People with Religious Convictions must know that Covid-19 vaccines may be contaminated with DNA from Aborted Babies

As of June 2020, thirty-three of the FDA approved vaccines on the market contain DNA fragments from various cell lines originating from aborted fetuses, where the virus is grown in the cell cultures derived from the tissues of those fetuses. Several of the Covid-19 vaccines have either used fetal cell lines in the development and/or production of the "vaccines" (gene therapy agents). And we are not talking about insignificant numbers of this human DNA in vaccines. In vaccines, the FDA allows 100,000,000 (yes one hundred million) bits and strands of human DNA per dose.

The leading vaccines (Covid-19) that involve the use of aborted fetal tissue are Moderna, Johnson & Johnson, AstraZeneca, Pfizer (used HEK-293 cells in testing). It is crucial that we fight for the right to oppose vaccines based on religious and medical exemptions. If we do not have freedom to choose what we put in our body, then what kind of freedom do we have left? We need to stand up and fight for our freedoms.

HUGE DAMAGE CAUSED BY COVID-19 VACCINES

The Covid-19 Plandemic was the biggest medical fraud of the decade. All the recommended measures to stop sickness were abject failure. Masks, sanitizers, social distancing, lockdowns, etc. were not only ineffective in reducing sickness but immensely disastrous to the natural health and immunity of the population. They also caused burden on the economy and proved to be an environmental hazard. The Covid-19 vaccine propaganda was pushed by the nexus of government, pharmaceuticals, politicians, media houses and medical establishments. Most of the people fell for the lies and took the experimental vaccine. This led to massive adverse reactions to millions of people across the world.

The Covid-19 vaccines were a brand-new gene therapy technology that were never tested or used in the human population. The clinical trials were cut short to get them to market in about 15% of the time typically required for new vaccines. There was no long-term safety data on them. The vaccine caused a terrifying and unprecedented number of reported serious adverse reactions and deaths. There was never a more orchestrated and aggressive push to get everyone vaccinated for anything in history.

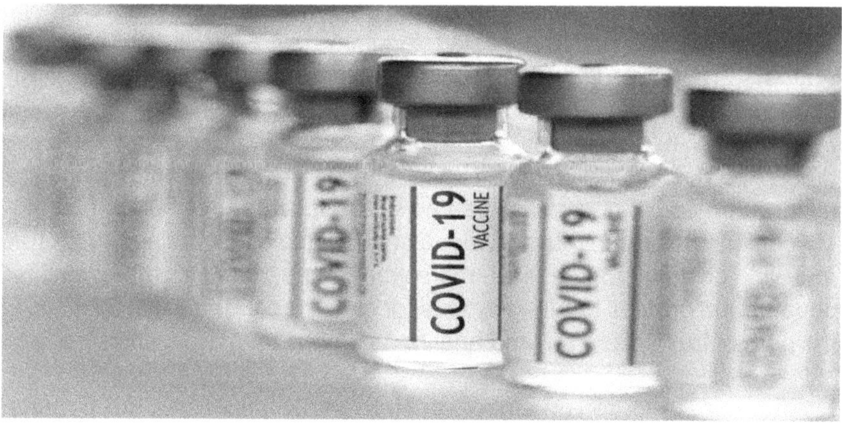

I have been informing the public about the vaccination agenda by the pharmaceutical companies from the beginning of 2020. It was similar to the previous medical frauds like HIV AIDS. The restrictions that were imposed on the population in the name of health were catastrophic. It made people submit to the unscientific, irrational, and harmful advice of the "medical experts". The masks did not stop or prevent a "viral" disease.

However, they were excellent for psychological operation on the minds of the population. Constant wearing of masks by every person portrayed the spread of a fatal disease and kept the fear instilled in every mind and heart. The sanitizers were harmful for natural immunity and skin health. The lockdowns were to keep the society disintegrated and shut down small businesses (and make them financially dependent on the government). Social distancing caused loneliness and alienation that led to high amounts of stress and harmed natural immunity. I have explained in detail with all top-grade evidence that masks, lockdowns, etc. were never proven to help the society in my book "Do Face Masks Really Work?".

The Covid-19 vaccine was completely ineffective in stopping or preventing cough, cold, diarrhea, etc. (so called symptoms of Covid-19). However, it had the potential to cause numerous side effects which took 9 pages for Pfizer to list together in a document titled Cumulative Analysis of Post-authorization Adverse Event Reports.[50] (See page no. 30 to 38)

The adverse reactions that people in my circle informed me included diabetes type-1, IBS, rheumatoid arthritis, thyroid malfunction, heart attacks, brain strokes, blood clots, hypertension, eczema, bell's palsy, miscarriage, chronic weakness, pneumonia, breathing difficulties, and even cardiac arrest (death).

For raising awareness on the above topics, I took to social media. I made videos, wrote articles, and posted regularly. As a result, my YouTube videos were deleted, and my channel was frozen multiple times. My Facebook account gets restricted multiple times. My Instagram account was shadow banned. My TikTok videos were removed and even my WhatsApp number was blocked once. I was vilified by some conventional (ignorant) medical doctors and some of the members of our community. My content was removed by various organisations that initially supported my work. Last but not the least, there were many threats from unidentified people. I am grateful to Almighty God for giving me the strength for walking the path of truth, freedom, and health.

I was fortunate to be a member of "Network of Influenza Care Experts" started by Dr. Biswaroop Roy Chowdhury to provide natural treatment for Covid-19 symptoms (an Influenza Like Illness) and dispel the misinformation campaigns by the medical establishment.[51] This team was successfully able to cure more than 60,000 patients diagnosed "positive" for Covid-19 by providing them natural immunity boosting protocol and helping manage the fear and stress. I was fortunate to serve and care for more than 250 people who had such symptoms.

Vaccine Adverse Event Reporting System (VAERS)

According to the VAERS, 27532 deaths and 152946 hospitalizations have been associated with Covid-19 vaccine as of April 2022. There have been 1,247,129 reported Covid-19 vaccine injuries in various categories of adverse events including myocarditis, thrombosis, heart attack, miscarriages, facial paralysis, permanent disability, and many more, in addition to the 27532 deaths. The death reports after Covid-19 vaccines are more than total deaths by all other vaccines combined over the last 30 years.[52] This is shocking! The chart below is the summary of the injuries:

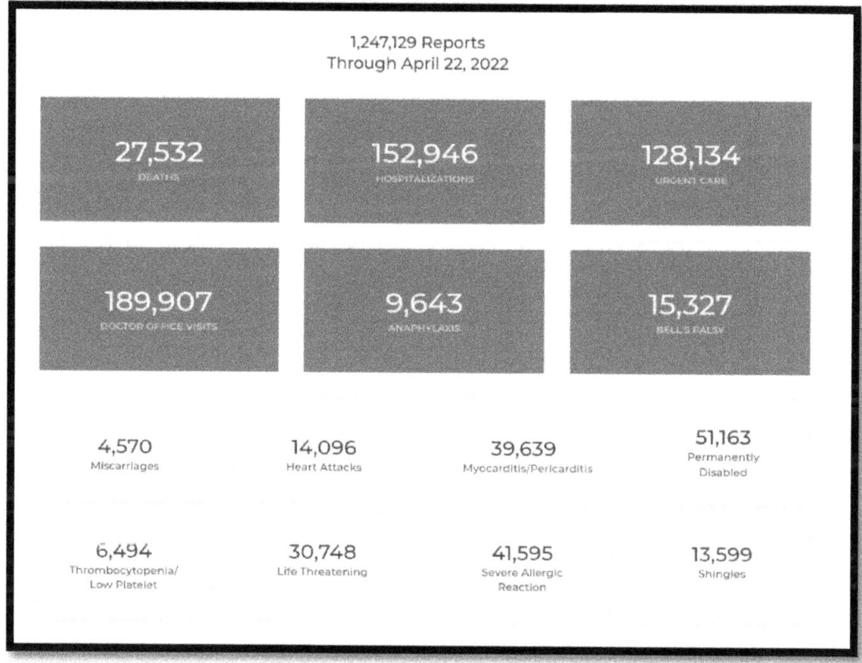

VAERS is a passive reporting system which means that vaccine reactions are not compulsory to be reported. It is completely voluntary and the person that has received the vaccine would have to know that it even exists and if they do how to report. Nearly all consumers and most doctors do not even know that a vaccine injury reporting system exists. Most of the people are not even able to draw the connection of their new disease and the vaccine because it was socially accepted that the vaccine was safe and effective despite the mountain of evidence showing that it can be extremely fatal in many cases.

This presents a problem of extreme under-reporting as verified by a U.S. government funded Harvard Pilgrim Health study that determined that less than 1% of all adverse vaccine reactions are reported to VAERS.[53]

Think about it for a minute. If less than 1% of the adverse reactions to vaccines are ever reported, what would you do to reach the actual figures? Add two zeros to the end of each of those numbers and it may be more representative of the actual numbers. You quickly realize that the 27,532 deaths become 2,753,200 deaths and so on.

If we consider that 10% percent of adverse reactions and deaths have been reported (instead of 1%) you would then add one zero to the reported deaths and the actual number would be 275,320 deaths associated with Covid-19 vaccine. Doesn't it seem frightening?

Why did Vaccine associated death statistics explode in 2021?

In the following table, you can see the number of deaths that are associated with vaccines every year. You can clearly see the number of vaccine associated deaths explode in 2021 (when covid-19 vaccines were rolled out).

Year	Deaths	Year	Deaths	Year	Deaths	Year	Deaths
1990	80	1998	172	2006	220	2014	358
1991	166	1999	179	2007	262	2015	377
1992	228	2000	212	2008	333	2016	437
1993	234	2001	225	2009	337	2017	467
1994	237	2002	187	2010	319	2018	535
1995	158	2003	265	2011	331	2019	604
1996	151	2004	208	2012	316	2020	421
1997	173	2005	215	2013	339	**2021**	**21884**

When the data of deaths associated with Covid-19 vaccine was analyzed, it was found that 3663 deaths happened within 24 hours of taking the vaccine, 2899 deaths happened within 48 hours of taking the vaccine and 1378 deaths happened in 72 hours of taking the vaccine.[52]

Ineffectiveness of Covid-19 vaccine was scientifically proven and published in 2021 in The Lancet – A top Medical Journal

Study title: COVID-19 vaccine efficacy and effectiveness – the elephant (not) in the room[54]; *The Lancet, July 2021*

Description: The Absolute Risk Reduction by any Covid-19 vaccine was only about 1% instead of 95% as claimed by vaccine manufacturers. Therefore, the vaccine might be 1% effective in preventing symptoms of Covid-19. Just 1%? That means after vaccinating 100 people, it will prevent infection in 1 person relatively. Quite useless!

Covid-19 Vaccine Increases the Miscarriage Risk by 50X

According to VAERS, 3429 miscarriages were reported in the year 2021.[52] In the following table, you can see the number of miscarriages (fetal deaths) that are associated with all vaccines every year. You can clearly see the number of vaccine associated miscarriages have exploded in 2021 (when covid-19 vaccines were rolled out on the mass population).

Year	Miscarriages	Year	Miscarriages	Year	Miscarriages
1990	05	1998	14	2006	51
1991	04	1999	06	2007	134
1992	06	2000	14	2008	224
1993	06	2001	23	2009	256
1994	05	2002	23	2010	235
1995	05	2003	28	2011	180
1996	19	2004	34	2012	120
1997	13	2005	25	2013	122

Year	Miscarriages
2014	90
2015	74
2016	59
2017	70
2018	79
2019	81
2020	65
2021	**3429**

The average miscarriage rate associated with vaccines per year was 67 per year. However, in 2021, the vaccine related miscarriages shot up to 3429. It shows a 50X increase in miscarriages caused by vaccines. The miscarriages caused by Covid-19 vaccine in 2021 alone is greater than the total miscarriages by all vaccines in the last 31 years. Isn't it shocking?

More than 20% women experienced irregular bleeding after the Covid-19 vaccine while 40% had menstrual changes

Study title: The effect of BNT162b2 SARS-CoV-2 mRNA vaccine on menstrual cycle symptoms in healthy women[56]; *International Journal of Gynecology & Obstetrics, July 2022*

Results from the study: "A total of 219 women met the inclusion criteria. Of them, 23.3% (n=51) experienced irregular bleeding following the vaccine. Almost 40% (n=83) of study participants reported any menstrual change following vaccination."

More than 20% people experienced Inflammatory Arthritis Symptoms after the Covid-19 vaccine

Study title: Incidence of Autoimmune Arthritis Disease Flare Following SARS-CoV-2 Vaccination and its Association with Concurrent NSAID Use[57]; *International Journal of Disease Reversal and Prevention, (2022)*

From the Study: This study aims to analyze the association between COVID-19 vaccination and an inflammatory arthritis reaction in autoimmune arthritis patients. A survey was completed by participants with inflammatory arthritis between August 17 and 18, 2021. Survey participants (n = 1348) responded to questions about their diagnosis, the length of their diagnosis, current medication, brand of vaccine received, incidence of inflammatory arthritis symptoms after COVID-19 vaccination, and how long the symptoms persisted. Following vaccination, 21% of participants reported experiencing inflammatory arthritis symptoms.

Covid-19 Vaccines Increase the Risk of Myocarditis by 4X

Study Title: SARS-CoV-2 vaccine and increased myocarditis mortality risk: A population based comparative study in Japan[55]; *MedArchive (2022)*

Conclusion: SARS-CoV-2 vaccination was associated with higher risk of myocarditis death, not only in young adults but also in all age groups including the elderly. The risk of myocarditis mortality in the SARS-CoV-2 vaccinated population may be 4 times or higher.

WHY ARE YOUNG AND FIT ATHLETES DYING SUDDENLY FROM CARDIAC ARRESTS?

There are three main mechanisms which can cause heart function to fail. One is due to blockage or obstruction in the arteries and veins to/from the heart. The second is cardiomyopathy, a disease or damage to the heart muscle. And the third is a malfunction of the heart's electrical system embedded in the heart. What is unusual and very concerning is that the increase in sudden deaths in fit and healthy young people is due to malfunction of the heart's electrical system. It is often triggered by an inflammatory condition, such as myocarditis.

1800% Increase in Sudden Deaths in 2021-22 in Athletes [146]

From Jan 2021 to Nov 2022, sudden deaths of 1101 athletes from cardiac arrests have been recorded – since the start of the mass Covid-19 injection campaign. The true death and injury numbers are likely to be much higher than what has been recorded as it is based on incidences being reported by members of the public. The dozens of other reports that are not or may not be vaccine-related have not been included.

Fit and healthy young people are suffering cardiac arrests at an alarming rate, yet corporate media and government won't discuss it. Cardiologists, physicians, doctors, and scientists around the world are greatly concerned about the alarming increase in cardiac arrests in fit, healthy people in the prime of their lives. Yet corporate media and an astonishing number of politicians refuse to acknowledge or discuss the harm and deaths caused by Covid injections. It is definitely not normal for so many mainly young athletes to suffer from cardiac arrests or to die while playing their sport, but this year it is happening.

Notably, in a 38-years timespan (1966-2004), 1101 athletes under the age of 35 died. It averages 29 deaths per year due to various heart-related conditions in athletes, 50% of who had congenital anatomical heart disease and cardiomyopathies and 10% had atherosclerotic heart disease with early onset.[147]

What that means is that normally in a period of about 38 years, about 1101 athletes would die from heart related complications. Which comes to an average of 29 deaths per year. However, in the period of 2021-22, we have seen 1101 athletes die from cardiac arrest. Which shows that after the rollout of covid-19 injections the death rate rose from 29 per year to 551 per year, showing a 1800% increase in death rate due to heart complications.

According to a study done on 301 teenagers between the ages of 13 and 18 who had received two doses of the Pfizer/BioNTech vaccine, 29.24% of participants experienced cardiovascular complications such tachycardia, palpitations and 2.33% suffered myopericarditis.[148] It shows that vaccinated people are at a much greater risk of heart related complications.

It is noteworthy, that no statistically significant increase in the incidence of myocarditis or pericarditis was observed in un-vaccinated subjects after SARS-CoV-2 infection, in a large population study.[149] It implies that myocarditis and heart complications are not a result of Covid-19 disease, but it is a result of the Covid-19 vaccine. Which implies that the current sudden cardiac arrest phenomenon is not prevalent in unvaccinated individuals.

Comment: If it was proven that the Covid-19 vaccine was highly ineffective and also unsafe, then why was it experimented on people on such a gigantic scale. The answer is to bring humanity into a New World Order which I have described in my book "Do Face Masks Really Work: An Introduction to the New World Order".

UNVACCINATED CHILDREN ARE HEALTHIER IN COMPARISON TO VACCINATED CHILDREN

For many years, vaccine educated people and organizations have been asking the CDC, WHO, pharmaceutical companies, and other relevant governmental agencies to do comparison studies looking at the health status, frequency of doctor's visits, and hospitalizations of children that have been vaccinated and those that have not been vaccinated. They have all refused to conduct such studies till now. Thankfully, recently some studies have been done by outstanding independent researchers who are not affiliated or supported by any of the organisations mentioned above. Here we look at some of those brilliant independent studies without conflict of interest and industry bias.

LATEST: A study published in November 2020 reveals that the children who never took any vaccine are much healthier than the children who took all the vaccines!

Study title: Relative Incidence of Office Visits and Cumulative Rates of Billed Diagnoses Along the Axis of Vaccination[58]; *International Journal of Environmental Research and Public Health, November 2020*

Description: This study categorizes the illnesses that vaccinated and unvaccinated children went for doctor's office visits during their first nine and a half years of life. It is a peer-reviewed study that shows clearly that unvaccinated children are healthier than vaccinated children.

From the Abstract: Increased office visits related to many diagnoses were robust to days-of-care-matched analyses, family history, gender block, age block, and false discovery risk. Many outcomes had high RIOV odds ratios after matching for days-of-care (e.g., anemia (6.334), asthma (3.496), allergic rhinitis (6.479), and sinusitis (3.529), all significant under the Z-test)."

"Remarkably, zero of the 561 unvaccinated patients in the study had attention deficit hyperactivity disorder (ADHD) compared to 0.063% of the (partially and fully) vaccinated. The implications of these results for the net public health effects of whole-population vaccination and with respect for informed consent on human health are compelling. Our results give agency to calls for research conducted by individuals who are independent of any funding sources related to the vaccine industry."

Conclusions of the study: "We could detect no widespread negative health effects in the vaccinated other than the rare but significant vaccine-targeted diagnosis. We can conclude that the unvaccinated children in this practice are not, overall, less healthy than the vaccinated and that indeed the vaccinated children appear to be significantly less healthy than the unvaccinated."

The following table shows the Relative Index of Office Visits for the fully vaccinated (N1 = 2763) vs. never vaccinated (N2 = 561).

Condition	Vaxxed	Unvaxxed	RIOV	95% CI	Z	p
Fever	759	17	9.065	8.801	12.476	<0.0001
"Well Child" Visits	32,826	4987	1.336	1.149	6.540	<0.0001
Ear Pain	269	16	3.414	3.232	5.310	<0.0001
Otitis media	3105	216	2.919	2.518	23.441	<0.0001
Conjunctivitis	1018	87	2.376	1.935	9.783	<0.0001
Eye Disorders (Other)	277	31	1.814	1.586	3.350	0.0008
Asthma	336	13	5.248	5.065	6.693	<0.0001
Allergic Rhinitis	405	12	6.853	6.662	8.158	<0.0001
Sinusitis	107	5	4.345	4.240	3.566	0.00036
Breathing Issues	621	44	2.866	2.561	7.898	<0.0001
Anemia	979	36	5.522	5.181	13.603	<0.0001
Eczema	512	23	4.520	4.281	8.479	<0.0001
Urticaria	174	17	2.078	1.908	3.027	0.00244
Dermatitis	742	105	1.435	0.992	4.034	<0.0001
Behavioral Issues	343	17	4.097	3.900	6.087	<0.0001
Gastroenteritis	688	30	4.656	4.374	6.543	<0.0001
Weight/Eating Disorders	1115	90	2.515	2.056	10.264	<0.0001
Seizure	43	8	1.091	0.985	0.229	0.8181

RIOVs were calculated using the number of patients as the sample size in each group (Vaxxed and Unvaxxed) with the exception of well-child visits and otitis media visits, both of which were greater in number than the number of patients.

What can we understand from the above table? The above table portrays that that the vaccinated group of children has relatively about 6 times more episodes of allergic rhinitis, about 5 times more episodes of asthma, about 5 times more episodes of anemia, about 4 times more episodes of sinusitis, about 4 times more episodes of eczema and about 9 times more episodes of fever besides increased risk of all other diseases like ear and eye disorders, stomach disorders, behaviour disorders, etc. It would not be wrong to say that Vaccinated children are sicker in all parameters as compared to children who never took any vaccines.

The graph on the next page displays the comparison of Visits to Doctors Office by children who are fully vaccinated and the children who never took any vaccines.

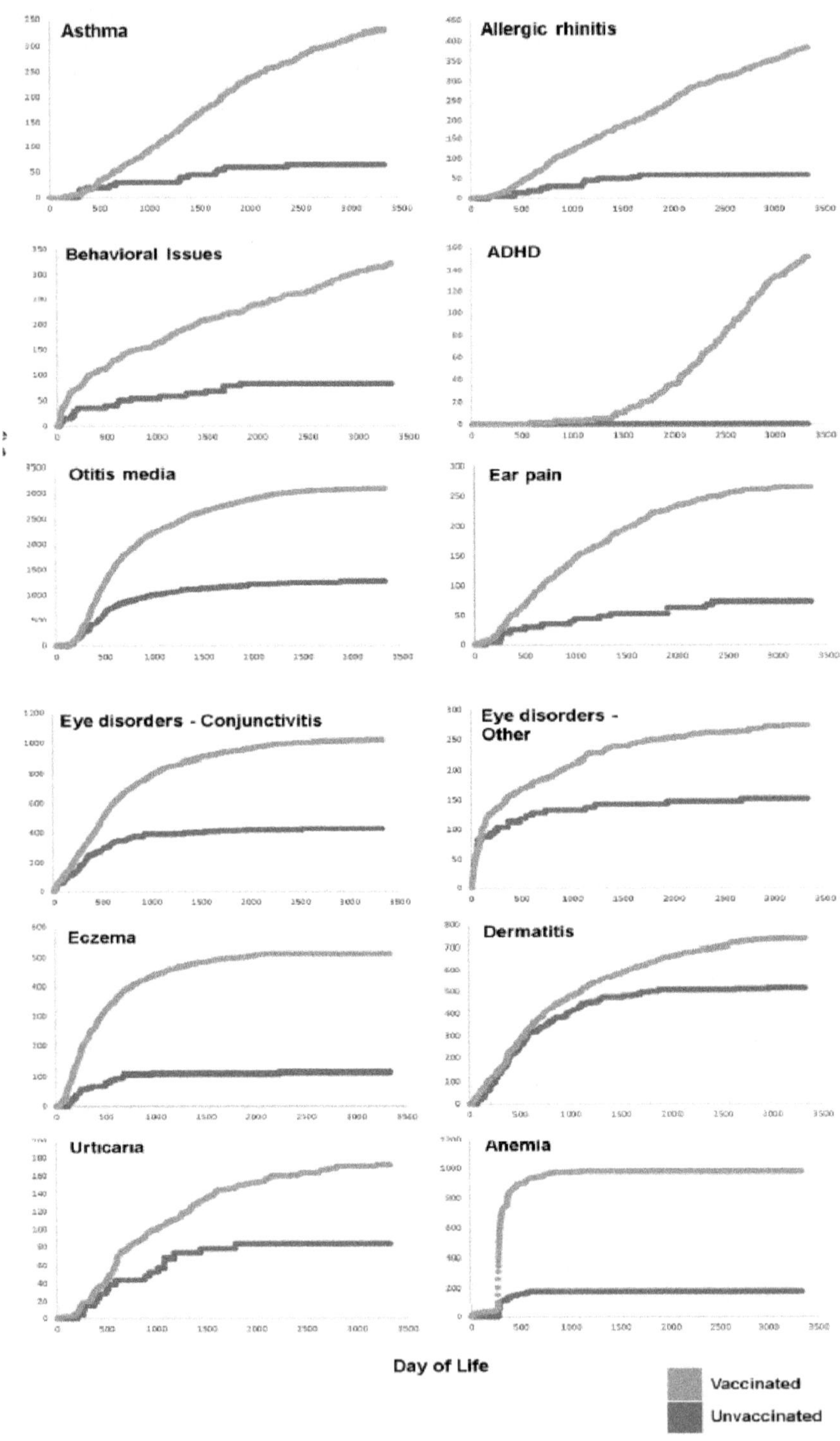
Asthma
Allergic rhinitis
Behavioral Issues
ADHD
Otitis media
Ear pain
Eye disorders - Conjunctivitis
Eye disorders - Other
Eczema
Dermatitis
Urticaria
Anemia
Day of Life
Vaccinated
Unvaccinated

What can we understand from the above graphs? The above graph visually displays that the fully vaccinated group of children had to make multiple times more office visits to the Doctor for all kinds of diseases. Now, who needs to make more visits to the doctor, the healthy person, or the sick person? The sick person! It shows multiple times more doctor visits for various health conditions are made by fully vaccinated group of children. The only conclusion one can draw from the above is that the unvaccinated children are much healthier than the fully vaccinated children.

Another landmark study comparing the health of vaccinated to unvaccinated children, shows superior health outcomes in the non-vaccinated group

Study title: Pilot comparative study on the health of vaccinated and unvaccinated 6-to 12-year-old U.S. children[59]; *Journal of Translational Science, April 2017*

Description: The study consisted of 666 children of which 261 (38%), were unvaccinated. The children were all between 6 and 12 years of age. Of the vaccinated group, 208 were partially and 197 fully vaccinated. Fully vaccinated is according to the full CDC schedule. Partially is anything less.

From the study: "Vaccinated children were significantly more likely than the unvaccinated to have been diagnosed with the following: allergic rhinitis (10.4% vs. 0.4%), other allergies (22.2% vs. 6.9%), eczema/atopic dermatitis (9.5% vs. 3.6%), a learning disability (5.7% vs. 1.2%), ADHD (4.7% vs. 1.0%), ASD (4.7% vs. 1.0%), any neurodevelopmental disorder (i.e., learning disability, ADHD or Autism Spectrum Disorder-ASD) (10.5% vs. 3.1%) and any chronic illness (44.0% vs. 25.0%)."

"The vaccinated (combining the partially and fully vaccinated) were significantly more likely than the unvaccinated to use medication for allergies (20.0% vs. 1.2%), to have used antibiotics in the past 12 months (30.8% vs. 15.4%), and to have used fever medications at least once (90.7% vs. 67.8%). The vaccinated were also more likely to have seen a doctor for a routine checkup in the past 12 months (57.6% vs. 37.2%), visited a dentist during the past year (89.4% vs. 80.5%), visited a doctor or clinic due to illness in the past year (36.0% vs. 16.0%), been fitted with ventilation ear tubes (3.0% vs. 0.4%), and spent one or more nights in a hospital (19.8% vs. 12.3%)."

MORE VACCINES LEAD TO MORE HOSPITALISATIONS MORE VACCINES LEAD TO MORE INFANT DEATHS

Multiple doses of vaccines in a single doctor visit increases the risk of health complications exponentially

Article title: Combining Childhood Vaccines at One Visit Is Not Safe[60]; *American Physicians and Surgeons, 2016*

More Vaccine Doses = More Hospitalizations

From the study: "Of the 38,801 VAERS reports that we analyzed, 969 infants received two vaccine doses prior to the adverse event and 107 of those infants were hospitalized: a hospitalization rate of 11%. Of 1,959 infants who received three vaccine doses prior to the adverse event, 243 of them required hospitalization: 12.4%. For four doses, 561 of 3,909 infants were hospitalized: 14.4%. Notice the emerging pattern: Infants who had an adverse event reported to VAERS were more likely to require hospitalization when they received three vaccine doses instead of two, or four vaccine doses instead of three."

Vaccine Doses	Hospitalised	Hospitalisation Rate
2	107/969	11%
3	243/1959	12.4%
4	561/3909	14.4%
5	1463/10114	14.5%
6	1365/8454	16.1%
7	1051/5489	19.1%
8	661/2817	23.5%

"The pattern continues: Of 10,114 infants who received five vaccine doses prior to the adverse event, 1,463 of them required hospitalization: 14.5%. For six doses, 1,365 of 8,454 infants were hospitalized: 16.1%. For seven doses, 1,051 of 5,489 infants were hospitalized: 19.1%. And for eight doses, 661 of 2,817 infants were hospitalized: 23.5%. The hospitalization rate increased linearly from 11.0% for two doses to 23.5% for eight doses."

More Vaccine Doses = More Mortality (here, 50% more death rate)

From the study: "Our study also calculated the case fatality ratio (mortality rate) among vaccinated infants, stratified by the number of vaccine doses they received. Of the 38,801 VAERS reports that we analyzed, 11,927 infants received one, two, three, or four vaccine doses prior to having an adverse event, and 423 of those infants died: a mortality rate of 3.6%. The remaining 26,874 infants received five, six, seven, or eight vaccine doses prior to the adverse event and 1,458 of them died: 5.4%. The mortality rate for infants who received five to eight vaccine doses (5.4%) is significantly higher than the mortality rate for infants who received one to four vaccine doses (3.6%)." "Of infants reported to VAERS, those who had received more vaccines had a statistically significant 50% higher mortality rate compared with those who had received fewer."

Vaccine Doses	Infants Died	Death Rate
1 to 4	423/11927	3.6%
5 to 8	1458/26874	5.4%

Conclusion of the study: The evidence presented in this study shows that multiple vaccines administered during one visit, and vaccinating young infants, significantly increase morbidity and mortality. Parents and physicians should consider health options associated with a lower risk of hospitalization or death."

Children who took more vaccines had to make more visits to the emergency department according to a study

Study title: A population-based cohort study of undervaccination in 8 managed care organizations across the United States[61]; *Journal of American Medical Association Pediatrics, March 2013*

Description: It analyzed 323,247 healthcare records to compare children under 2 years of age who were fully vaccinated at CDC-recommended ages to children who were under-vaccinated (they did not receive all vaccines according to the recommended schedule).

Comments: Children who were under-vaccinated had the greatest reductions in outpatient visits and healthcare utilization for upper respiratory illness, fever and pharyngitis when compared to on-time, fully vaccinated children (36% to 38% reductions).

Children who were under-vaccinated because of parental choice had lower inpatient admission rates and significantly lower rates of outpatient and emergency department visits (incidence rate ratio, IRR = 0.94 and 0.91, respectively) compared to on-time, fully vaccinated children.

Correlation of Infant Mortality Rates and Vaccine Doses

In 2009, the U.S. had the highest number of vaccine doses and was 34th in infant mortality rate. In 2009, the U.S. had the highest vaccine rate and 33 other nations had better infant (<1 year-old) mortality rates.

Study title: Infant mortality rates regressed against number of vaccine doses routinely given: is there a biochemical or synergistic toxicity?[62] *Human and Experimental Toxicology, September 2011*

From the study: "The US childhood immunization schedule specifies 26 vaccine doses for infants aged less than 1 year—the most in the world—yet 33 nations have lower IMRs." "Linear regression analysis of unweighted mean IMRs showed a high statistically significant correlation between increasing number of vaccine doses and increasing infant mortality rates" "These findings demonstrate a counter-intuitive relationship: nations that require more vaccine doses tend to have higher infant mortality rates."

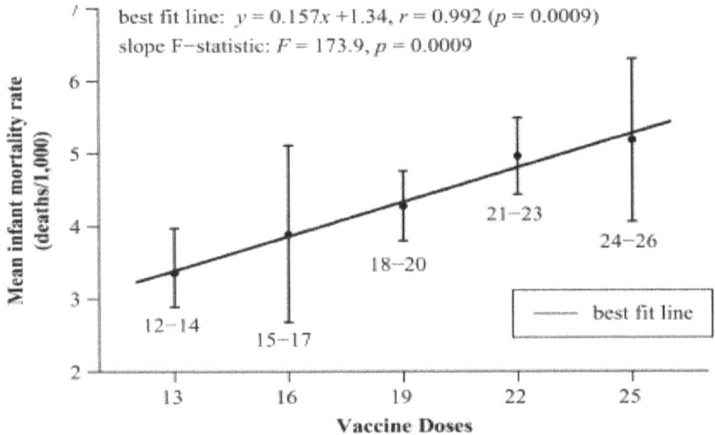

What can we understand from the above graph? It is clearly visible that the direct correlation between the number of doses of vaccines given and the proportional rising rate of infant mortality. The article also refers to previous studies that show a possible link between some cases of Sudden Infant Death (SIDS) and vaccination, specifically the DPT vaccine.

Comment: Sweden has the lowest number of doses of vaccines (12) given before age 1 and at the same time it has the lowest infant mortality rate (2009 statistics). The US ranked 34th and had the highest infant mortality rate along with the greatest number of vaccinations (26) given by age 1.

Japan Leads the Way: No Vaccine Mandates and No MMR Vaccine = Healthier Children in Japan

In another related story, this is the headline of a 2019 article on the Children's Health Defense website. It contrasts the dreadful infant mortality rate of the U.S. with Japan.[63]

From the article: "The U.S. has the very highest infant mortality rate of all industrialized countries, with more American children dying at birth and in their first year than in any other comparable nation — and more than half of those who survive develop at least one chronic illness."

The CDC views infant mortality as one of the most important indicators of a society's overall health. The agency should take note of Japan's rate, which, at 2 infant deaths per 1,000 live births, is the second lowest in the world. In comparison, almost three times as many American infants die (5.8 per 1,000 live births), despite massive per capita spending on health care for children. U.S. infant mortality ranks behind 55 other countries and is worse than the rate in Latvia, Slovakia, or Cuba. Here are key differences between the Japanese and U.S. vaccine programs:

"Unlike Japan, the U.S. administers flu and Tdap vaccines to pregnant women (during any trimester) and babies receive flu shots at six months of age, continuing every single year thereafter. Manufacturers have never tested the safety of flu shots administered during pregnancy, and the FDA has never formally licensed any vaccines specifically for use during pregnancy to protect the infant."

Question: If vaccines save lives, why are American children (who receive the maximum vaccine doses in the world) dying younger at a faster rate compared to children in 19 other wealthy countries — translating into a 57 percent greater risk of death before reaching adulthood?

SUDDEN INFANT DEATH SYNDROME: THE VACCINE CONNECTION

Sudden Infant Death (S.I.D.S.), SIDS is defined as "the sudden death of an infant under one year of age which remains unexplained after a thorough case investigation, including performance of a complete autopsy, death scene investigation, and review of the clinical history."

The connection of Haemophilus Influenza Type B (HIB) vaccine and Sudden Infant Death Syndrome

Study title: Adverse events following Haemophilus influenzae type b vaccines in the Vaccine Adverse Event Reporting System, 1990-2013[64]; *The Journal of Pediatrics, April 2015*

Results from the study: "VAERS received 29,747 reports after Hib vaccines; 5179 (17%) were serious, including 896 reports of deaths. Median age was 6 months (range 0-1022 months). Sudden infant death syndrome was the stated cause of death in 384 (51%) of 749 death reports with autopsy/death certificate records. The most common nondeath serious AE categories were neurologic (80; 37%), other non-infectious (46; 22%) (comprising mainly constitutional signs and symptoms); and gastrointestinal (39; 18%) conditions".

Comments: Considering that only 1-10% of adverse reactions are even reported to VAERS, even taking the more conservative 10% reporting into consideration, it would mean that 3,840 of the 8,960 reported deaths were classified as SIDS deaths during this period.

Sudden Infant Death Syndrome (SIDS) increases 13 times after the introduction of the Hexavalent Vaccine (6 vaccine combo)

Study title: Unexplained cases of sudden infant death shortly after hexavalent vaccination[65]; *Vaccine, 2006*

From the study: "We report six cases of sudden infant death after hexavalent vaccination that were autopsied and examined at the Munich Institute of Legal Medicine from 2001 to 2004." "Among those investigated children, three were male and three females, ageing between 4 and 17 months. Five children had been vaccinated with Hexavac®, one with Infanrix Hexa® during the past 48 hours before death. Shortly after the vaccination, three of the children developed symptoms like tiredness, loss of appetite, fever up to 39 ◦C and insomnia. All children were found dead without explanation 1–2 days after the vaccination."

"In addition to neuropathologic and histologic abnormalities, all of these children showed an extraordinary brain edema, which made them exceptional to other SID cases." "Prior to the release of hexavalent sera (in the years 1994–2000), we observed only one child out of 198 cases with sudden unexplained infant death who died shortly after vaccination (DTP). However, between 2001 and 2004 five of such cases were identified in our institution among 74 children with SID. This would indicate a 13-fold increase (the local autopsy rate for infants is about 70%)."

S.I.D.S. increased 30 times after vaccination with Hexavalent vaccine (6 in 1 combo) according to another study

Study title: Sudden and unexpected deaths after the administration of hexavalent vaccines (diphtheria, tetanus, pertussis, poliomyelitis, hepatitis B, Haemophilius influenzae type b): is there a signal?[66] *European Journal of Pediatrics, February 2005*

Description: This study finds that the hexavalent vaccine given in the second year of life caused mortality rates (death rates) on the first day after vaccination that were 31.3 times greater than national vital statistics rates! Sudden unexpected death (SUD) rate on the second day after vaccination were 23.5 times greater than the national rates!

EPIDEMIC OF AUTISM: THE VACCINE CONNECTION

In 1970, Treffert et. al. published the first known autism prevalence study in the United States, Epidemiology of Infantile Autism[67], with an autism prevalence rate of less than 1 per 10,000.

In 1987, Burd et. al. published a study, A prevalence study of pervasive developmental disorders in North Dakota, showing an autism rate of 3.3 per 10,000.[68]

In 2002, the Data & Statistics on Autism Spectrum Disorder by CDC shows that prevalence of autism had grown to 66 per 10,000.[69] It means 1 in 150 children will develop autism. It is an increase of more than 6,000% from the 1970 study.

In 2018, the Data & Statistics on Autism Spectrum Disorder by CDC shows that prevalence of autism had grown to 230 per 10,000.[69] It means 1 in 44 children will develop autism.

At the currently increasing rates of autism, some experts estimate that 1 in 2 children would be autistic by 2032!

Year	Autism Rate
1970	1 in 10,000
1987	1 in 3,000
2002	1 in 150
2018	1 in 44
2022	?

If 1 in 44 children were diagnosed with autism in 2018, then what would be the number now? And what would be the number after ten years? It is extremely frightening! Also, it is important to consider that these statistics do not cover many other developmental, neurological (like ADHD) and immunological effects (like allergies, asthma, and autoimmune disorders) that are now being associated with vaccine injury in the scientific literature. Just think about the cumulative effect personally and economically of the dramatic rise in prevalence of all these conditions! This rise in autism prevalence is highly co-related with the increasing doses of vaccines.

DOSES of VACCINES for U.S. CHILDREN from BIRTH-18 YEARS

1983

DTP (2 months)
OPV (2 months)
DTP (4 months)
OPV (4 months)
DTP (6 months)
MMR (15 months)
DTP (18 months)
OPV (18 months)
DTP (4 years)
OPV (4 years)
Td (15 years)

*1986:
Pharmaceutical manufacturers producing vaccines were freed from ALL liability resulting from vaccine injury or death by the Childhood Vaccine Injury Act.

2020

Influenza (Pregnancy)
TdaP (Pregnancy)
Hep B (birth)
Hep B (2 months)
Rotavirus (2 months)
DTaP (2 months)
HIB (2 months)
PCV (2 months)
IPV (2 months)
Rotavirus (4 months)
DTaP (4 months)
HIB (4 months)
PCV (4 months)
IPV (4 months)
Hep B (6 months)
Rotavirus (6 months)
DTaP (6 months)
HIB (6 months)
PCV (6 months)
IPV (6 months)
Influenza (6 months)
Influenza (7 months)
HIB (12 months)
PCV (12 months)
MMR (12 months)
Varicella (12 months)
Hep A (12 months)
DTaP (18 months)
Influenza (18 months)
Hep A (18 months)
Influenza (30 months)
Influenza (42 months)
DTaP (4 years)
IPV (4 years)
MMR (4 years)
Varicella (4 years)
Influenza (5 years)
Influenza (6 years)
Influenza (7 years)
Influenza (8 years)
Influenza (9 years)
Influenza (10 years)
HPV (11 years)
HPV (11 years)
Influenza (11 years)
TdaP (12 years)
Influenza (12 years)
Meningococcal (12 yrs)
Influenza (13 years)
Influenza (14 years)
Influenza (15 years)
Influenza (16 years)
Meningococcal (16 yrs)
Influenza (17 years)
Influenza (18 years)

2020
TOTAL DOSES: 69
Injections: 50
(3 Doses of Rotavirus are liquid)
1983
TOTAL DOSES: 24
Injections: 7
(4 Doses of Polio were liquid)

(SOURCE: www.cdc.gov)

DTP- Diphtheria, Tetanus, Pertussis (whole cell)
OPV- Oral Polio
MMR- Measles, Mumps, Rubella
Hep B- Hepatitis B
DTaP- Diphtheria, Tenatus, Pertussis (acellular)
HIB- Haemophilus influenzae Type B
PCV- Pneumococcal
IPV- Inactivated Polio
Varicella- Chicken Pox
Td- Tetanus, Diphtheria
Tdap- Tetanus, Diphtheria, and Pertussis
HPV- Human papillomavirus (Gardasil)

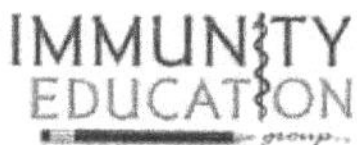

A report published in 2009 compared the vaccine doses, autism rates and infant mortality rates of US with 29 other countries and the results are extremely shocking

Study title: Autism and Vaccines Around the World: Vaccine Schedules, Autism Rates, and Under 5 Mortality[70]; *Generation Rescue, Inc. April 2009*

Results of the report: "The United States mandates the most vaccines in the Western world (36), double the average of the 30 countries studied (18). All countries with lower vaccine mandates have better under 5 mortality rates and many have materially lower autism rates."

TABLE 2: NUMBER OF MANDATORY VACCINES AND UNDER 5 MORTALITY RATES FOR TOP 30 COUNTRIES

Country	# of Mandatory Vaccines (<5 yrs old)	Mortality Rates Per 1,000 children Under 5 yrs old[i]	Mortality Rate Worldwide Rank
United States	**36**	**7.8**	**34**
Iceland	11	3.9	1
Sweden	11	4.0	2
Singapore	13	4.1	3
Japan	11	4.2	4
Norway	13	4.4	5
Finland	12	4.7	6
Hong Kong	13	4.7	7
Czech Republic	20	4.8	8
Korea, South	n.a.	4.8	9
Switzerland	16	5.1	10
France	17	5.2	11
Spain	20	5.3	12
Belgium	18	5.3	13
Germany	22	5.4	14
Austria	19	5.4	15
Australia	27	5.6	16
Israel	11	5.7	17
Denmark	12	5.8	18
Netherlands	20	5.9	19
Canada	28	5.9	20
United Kingdom	20	6.0	21
Italy	13	6.1	22
Ireland	24	6.2	23
Channel Islands	n.a.	6.2	24
Slovenia	14	6.4	25
New Zealand	21	6.4	26
Cuba	n.a.	6.5	27
Luxembourg	23	6.6	28
Portugal	19	6.6	29
Brunei	n.a.	6.7	30
Cyprus	23	6.9	31
Malta	14	7.6	32
Croatia	18	7.7	33
Average	**18.0**		

What can we understand from the above table? This table makes it clear that children in US receive the maximum number of vaccines (36) as compared to all other nations. And interestingly, US has the highest mortality rate in children (7.8) amongst them.

TABLE 3: VACCINE SCHEDULES, AUTISM RATES, AND UNDER 5 MORTALITY FOR SELECT COUNTRIES

Country	# of Mandatory Vaccines (<5 yrs old)	Autism Rate	US Autism Rate Multiplier	Mortality Rates Per 1,000 children Under 5 years old	Mortality Rate Worldwide Rank
United States	36	1 in 150		7.8	34
Iceland	11	1 in 1,100 [ii]	7.3 x	3.9	1
Sweden	11	1 in 862 [iii]	5.7 x	4.0	2
Japan	11	1 in 475 [iv]	3.2 x	4.2	4
Norway	13	1 in 2,000 [v]	13.3 x	4.4	5
Finland	12	1 in 719 [vi]	4.8 x	4.7	6
France	17	1 in 613 [vii]	4.1 x	5.2	11
Israel	11	1 in 1,000 [viii]	6.7 x	5.7	17
Denmark	12	1 in 2,200 [ix]	14.6 x	5.8	18

What can we understand from the above table? The table shows data from 2009 report. It reveals that The United States has the highest number of mandated vaccines of any country in the world (36) and at the same time it is the highest prevalence of autism in the world (1 in 150 children).

Vaccinated children have a 41% greater incidence of autism in comparison to unvaccinated children

Study title: Empirical Data Confirm Autism Symptoms Related to Aluminum and Acetaminophen Exposure[71]; *Entropy 2012*

From the article: "One can compute a 41% increased relative frequency of autism diagnosis in the vaccinated versus the unvaccinated population". "Finally, It is likely that other vaccines in addition to MMR play a role in autism". "MMR is often administered simultaneously with Diphtheria, Tetanus and Pertussis (DTaP), an aluminum-containing vaccine. The synergistic and cumulative effects of multiple vaccines would likely lead to nonlinear enhancement of adverse events."

MMR Vaccine is associated with Autism Spectrum Disorder (This vaccine is produced in aborted fetal cell lines)

A Natural Experiment: Rate of Autism dropped as MMR vaccine compliance rates dropped and as MMR vaccine compliance rates increased again, so did rates of autism. It shows a positive relation with MMR vaccine uptake and autism rates.

Study title: Epidemiologic and Molecular Relationship Between Vaccine Manufacture and Autism Spectrum Disorder Prevalence[48]; *Issues in Law and Medicine, 2015*

It was found out that the average MMR vaccine coverage for the three countries (United Kingdom, Norway, and Sweden) fell below 90% in 1998 till 2000. At the same time, the cases of autism also started reducing in those countries. Gradually, as the vaccine coverage started increasing again from 2001 and reached over 90% coverage again by 2004. At the same time, the cases of autism also started increasing in those countries. It clearly demonstrates that the MMR vaccine (and its ingredients) plays a role in causing autism spectrum disorder.

Researchers cite strong evidence of a connection between aluminum in vaccines and autism

Study title: Empirical Data Confirm Autism Symptoms Related to Aluminum and Acetaminophen Exposure[71]; *Entropy 2012*

From the study: "For each 1% increase in vaccination rate, 680 additional children were diagnosed with autism or speech delay." "All of the significant symptoms in the table—macule, cellulitis, blister, seizure, abscess, death, and low appetite—are also significant symptoms associated with the vaccines containing aluminum. This result further supports the possibility that the aluminum in these vaccines administered to young children may be even more toxic than the mercury." "This strong association does not however exclude mercury as a contributor to autism, given that Hep B has both mercury and aluminum. In fact, mercury and aluminum together may be synergistically toxic."

The acetaminophen (paracetamol) connection with autism

A growing body of evidence over the last 5-7 years suggests that the use of acetaminophen (i.e., Tylenol), blocks the body's ability to produce glutathione, which is considered the body's "Master Antioxidant". This also happens to a greater degree in genetically susceptible children that further prevents their bodies from eliminating toxins like mercury, aluminum, and other toxic substances in vaccines. It is not the acetaminophen that causes autism, rather its use in proximity to vaccination that appears to handcuff the body's ability to clear the metals and toxins.

While it is true that many children that regress into autism do so without having been given this drug, it now appears that the drug may significantly increase that risk.

Article title: Evidence that Increased Acetaminophen use in Genetically Vulnerable Children Appears to be a Major Cause of the Epidemics of Autism, Attention Deficit with Hyperactivity, and Asthma[72]; *William Shaw, November 2015*

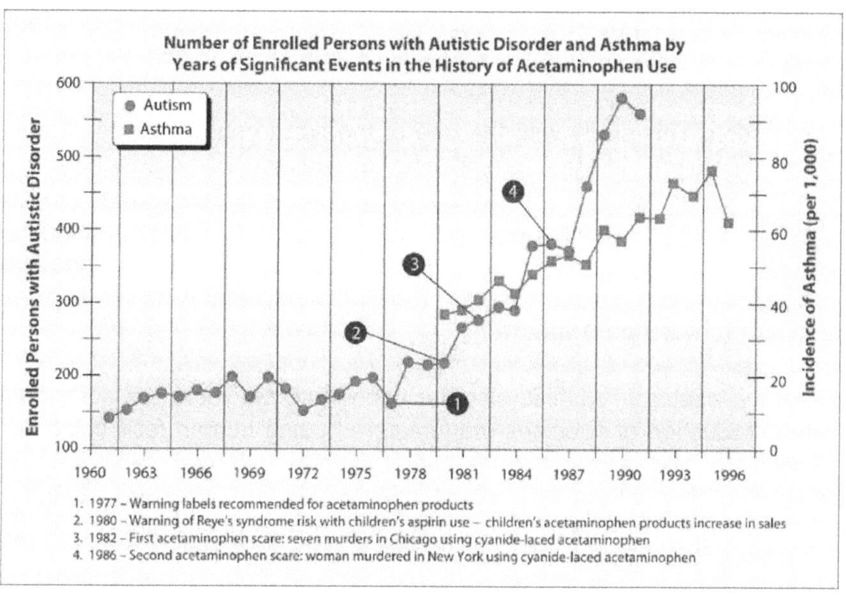

What can we understand from this graph? It shows that when the use of paracetamol increased, the cases of autism also increased. It also shows that when the use of paracetamol decreased, the cases of autism and asthma also decreased. It shows that paracetamol is another toxic drug that may increase the incidence of toxic accumulations in the body.

Some of the points on paracetamol mentioned in the discussed article are:

- Neurotoxic effects on brain neurons
- Maternal use during pregnancy is associated with teratogenic defects
- Severe immune abnormalities and immune response depression
- The leading cause of liver failure in the United States
- 56,000 emergency room visits in the US per year
- Increased rates of certain blood cancers

VACCINES PRODUCED WITH ABORTED FETAL CELLS ARE HIGHLY CONNECTED TO AUTISM

The increased rates of autism correlate with the inclusion of aborted human fetal cell lines and retroviruses into vaccines

Study name: Impact of Environmental Factors on the Prevalence of Autistic Disorder after 1979[73]; *Public Health and Epidemiology, September 2014*

Description: This study was the one of the first to show significant data point increases in the prevalence of autism corresponding with introduction of fetal cell line tissues and retroviruses into vaccines in the U.S. The same correlation was also found in the U.K., Western Australia, and Denmark when those elements were introduced. The vaccines that added these fetal tissues were the MMR, the Hepatitis A and B, and the Varicella (chickenpox) vaccine.

From the abstract: "Autistic disorder change points years are coincident with introduction of vaccines manufactured using human fetal cell lines, containing fetal and retroviral contaminants, into childhood vaccine regimens. This pattern was repeated in the US, UK, Western Australia, and Denmark. Thus, rising autistic disorder prevalence is directly related to vaccines manufactured utilizing human fetal cells."

From the study: "In 1979, coincident with the first autism disorder change point, vaccine manufacturing changes introduced human fetal DNA fragments and retroviral contaminants into childhood vaccines (Victoria et al., 2010). While we do not know the causal mechanism behind these new vaccine contaminants and autistic disorder, human fetal DNA fragments are inducers of autoimmune reactions, while both DNA fragments and retroviruses are known to potentiate genomic insertions and mutations (Yolken et al., 2000; Kurth 1998; U S Food and Drug Administration 2011"

Comments: The spikes in autism produced what is called a hockey stick appearance with a steep increase starting at the time of introduction of these cells which can be seen in the graphs on page 4 of the article.

VACCINES MAY CAUSE AUTISM, BRAIN DAMAGE AND OTHER NEUROLOGICAL DISORDERS

Vaccines with aluminum adjuvants can compromise brain development and cause permanent neurological impairments

Book Section title: Autism Spectrum Disorders and Aluminum Vaccine Adjuvants[74]; *A Comprehensive Guide to Autism*

From the Abstract: "Impaired brain function, excessive inflammation, and autoimmune manifestations are common in autism. Aluminum (Al), the most commonly used vaccine adjuvant, is a demonstrated neurotoxin and a strong immune stimulator. Hence, adjuvant Al has the necessary properties to induce neuroimmune disorders". "In summary, research data suggests that vaccines containing Al may be a contributing etiological factor in the increasing incidence of autism."

Vaccines with thimerosal are linked to neurological disorders

Study title: Low-dose Thimerosal in pediatric vaccines: Adverse effects in perspective[75]; *Environmental Research, January 2017*

From the article: "Thimerosal, known to have neurotoxic effects even at low doses, has not been scrutinized for the limit of tolerance alone or in combination with adjuvant - Al during immaturity or developmental periods (pregnant women, newborns, infants, and young children). "However, consistently, they showed a link of EtHg with risk of certain neurodevelopment disorders, such as tic disorder, while clearly revealing the benefits of removing Thimerosal from children's vaccines (associated with immunological reactions) in developed countries." "The collective evidence strongly suggests that Thimerosal exposure is associated with adverse neurodevelopmental outcomes."

Evidence suggests that mercury (a vaccine ingredient) can cause brain damage and lead to autism spectrum disorders

Study title: A comprehensive review of mercury provoked autism[76]; *Indian Journal of Medical Research, October 2008*

From the article: “Emerging evidence supports the theory that some autism spectrum disorders (ASDs) may result from a combination of genetic/biochemical susceptibility, specifically a reduced ability to excrete mercury (Hg), and exposure to Hg at critical developmental periods.” “In conclusion, the overwhelming preponderance of the evidence favours acceptance that Hg exposure is capable of causing some ASDs.”

A study involving nearly 300,000 children, found “consistent significantly increased” rates of autism, ADD and emotional disturbances linked to Thimerosal Containing Vaccines (TCVs)

Study title: Thimerosal exposure in infants and neurodevelopmental disorders: an assessment of computerized medical records in the Vaccine Safety Datalink[77]; *Journal of the Neurological Sciences, August 2008*

From the article: “Consistent significantly increased rate ratios were observed for autism, autism spectrum disorders, tics, attention deficit disorder, and emotional disturbances with Hg exposure from Thimerosal Containing Vaccines.” “Efforts should be undertaken to remove Hg from vaccines.”

Using data from U.S. Government records, a 2004 study finds a strong correlation with levels of mercury from vaccines and rates of autism.

Study title: A comparative evaluation of the effects of MMR immunization and mercury doses from thimerosal-containing childhood vaccines on the population prevalence of autism[78]; *Medical Science Monitor, March 2004*

From the study: “These studies have shown that there is biological plausibility and epidemiological evidence showing a direct relationship between increasing doses of mercury from thimerosal-containing vaccines and neurodevelopmental disorders, and measles-containing vaccines and serious neurological disorders. It is recommended that thimerosal be removed from all vaccines.”

ALUMINUM IN VACCINES IS POISONOUS: MAY LEAD TO NEUROLOGICAL DISORDERS AND INCREASE RISKS OF ALZHEIMERS DISEASE

Aluminum exposure from vaccines, causes a wide array of neurological and autoimmune disorders including autism

Study title: Aluminum in the central nervous system (CNS): toxicity in humans and animals, vaccine adjuvants, and autoimmunity[79]; *Immunologic Research, July 2013*

From the abstract: "In young children, a highly significant correlation exists between the number of pediatric aluminum-adjuvanted vaccines administered and the rate of autism spectrum disorders. Many of the features of aluminum-induced neurotoxicity may arise, in part, from autoimmune reactions, as part of the ASIA syndrome."

Seven childhood vaccines containing aluminum, some given together in multiple doses called out as a high risk for toxicity

Study title: The meaning of aluminium exposure on human health and aluminium-related diseases[80]; *Biomolecular Concepts, February 2013*

From the study: "Aluminium is unquestionably neurotoxic, as has been well demonstrated in multiple experimental animals and in clinical practice." "Aluminium is used as an adjuvant in multiple childhood vaccines, including DtaP, Pediatrix (DtaP, hepatitis B, polio combination), Pentacel (DtaP, HIB, polio combination), hepatitis A, hepatitis B, Haemophilus influentiza B (HIB), human papilloma virus (HPV) and pneumococcal vaccines." "Taken all together, these data clearly indicate that aluminium represents a significant component of exposure of humans to xenobiotics and contaminants and that newborns are at risk of aluminium-related toxicity not only in the perinatal period, but also in childhood and in adulthood"

Current research implicates long-term, low-level aluminum exposure as one of the main causes of early brain aging and age-related neurological diseases

Study title: Prolonged exposure to low levels of aluminum leads to changes associated with brain aging and neurodegeneration[81]; *Toxicology, January 2014*

Description: The study correlated long-term low-level exposure of aluminum, which is what we are exposed to with vaccines to brain aging and neurodegeneration. Currently there are 26 vaccines marketed in the U.S. that contain aluminum.

From the article: "Epidemiological studies suggest that aluminum may not be as innocuous as was previously thought and that aluminum may actively promote the onset and progression of Alzheimer's disease. Epidemiological data is strengthened by experimental evidence of aluminum exposure leading to excess inflammatory activity within the brain." "Evidence is outlined supporting the concept of aluminum's involvement in hastening brain aging. This acceleration would then inevitably lead to increased incidence of specific age-related neurological diseases."

2017 study from the journal Metabolic Brain Disease calls for the phase out of aluminum adjuvants ASAP

Study title: The putative role of environmental aluminium in the development of chronic neuropathology in adults and children. How strong is the evidence and what could be the mechanisms involved?[82] *Metabolic Brain Disease, October 2017*

Description: The study finds serious problems with the continued use of aluminum adjuvants in vaccines and the risk it exposes to pregnant women, women planning on becoming pregnant and children.

From the conclusions: "Aluminium has no known beneficial physiological action in the human body and some genetic polymorphisms predispose to a greater susceptibility to its adverse effects. Therefore, a strong case can be made for avoiding unnecessary exposure to environmental sources of aluminium salts, especially on the part of children, pregnant mothers, and women of child - bearing age who may become pregnant." "It would seem prudent to try to find an alternative to aluminium adjuvants as soon as possible and phase out their use."

Intravenous aluminum impacts mental development scores

Study title: Aluminum Neurotoxicity and Preterm Infants Receiving Intravenous Feeding Solutions[83]; *New England Journal of Medicine, May 1997*

From the article: "The former (the group with standard levels of 25 mcg/dl aluminum in the feeding solution), were significantly more likely (39 percent, vs. 17 percent of the latter group) to have a Mental Development Index of less than 85, increasing their risk of subsequent educational problems. For all 157 infants without neuromotor impairment, increasing aluminum exposure was associated with a reduction in the Mental Development Index, with an adjusted loss of one point per day of intravenous feeding for infants receiving the standard solutions." "In infants fed intravenously for 10 or more days, those receiving the standard solutions had a major (10 point) deficit in their Mental Development Index and were twice as likely to have a Mental Development Index below 85." "Intravenous aluminum may have neurotoxic effects, longer-term consequences for neurologic development."

Conclusions: "In preterm infants, prolonged intravenous feeding with solutions containing aluminum is associated with impaired neurologic development."

Comments: To be clear, vaccines are delivered by injection and there is no reason to believe that the results would be any different than in this study. As many studies in this document reveal, metals travel from the injection site to distant parts of the body, including the organs and brain.

There are huge amounts of aluminum in childhood vaccines!

At birth, most children are given the hepatitis B vaccination which has 250 mcg. of aluminum.[84] This is almost 10x the amount of aluminum that is approved by FDA. It gets much worse as multiple vaccines containing high levels of aluminum are piled on. The total amount of aluminum given to children in routine vaccines by age 18 months, is approximately 100 times greater than the daily amount deemed safe intravenously by the FDA for an average size baby at 23 pounds. While it is true that the aluminum is given in "batches" throughout that 18 month as reported above, sometimes those batches include up to 1,000 mcg at a time. And all the while, more and more are being stored in the brain and other organs. This can be catastrophic!

So, we learn from FDA documents that if a premature baby receives more than 10 mcg of aluminum in an IV, it can accumulate in their bones and brain, and can be toxic. The FDA maximum restrictions for aluminum received in an IV is 25 mcg. The suggested aluminum per kg (2.2 pounds), of weight to give to a person is up to 5 mcg/day. (So, a 5-pound baby should get no more than 11 mcg of aluminum.) All I.V. products given for parenteral nutrition are required to contain less than 25 mcg of aluminum. In addition, all products are to have a warning on the label that reads:

"WARNING: This product contains aluminum that may be toxic. Aluminum may reach toxic levels with prolonged parenteral administration if kidney function is impaired. Premature neonates are particularly at risk because their kidneys are immature, and they require large amounts of calcium and phosphate solutions, which contain aluminum.[85]

Research indicates that patients with impaired kidney function, including premature neonates, who receive parenteral levels of aluminum at greater than 4 to 5 mcg per kg per day accumulate aluminum at levels associated with central nervous system and bone toxicity. Tissue loading may occur at even lower rates of administration."

Note: Vaccines, for some reason, are not required to have this label and also are not required to follow the maximum dosage of 25 mcg.

All of the vaccines and direct access to their package inserts containing all the ingredients including aluminum levels can be found here: http://www.immunize.org/fda/

THIMEROSAL IN VACCINES IS POISONOUS: MAY LEAD TO REPRODUCTIVE ISSUES AND INCREASE IN RISK OF PREMATURE PUBERTY

Thimerosal is proven to be toxic even at minute levels, but it is still present in vaccines given to pregnant women and children

While it is true that thimerosal has been removed from most childhood vaccines, the industry is still pushing the flu and Tdap vaccines on pregnant women, when the baby in-utero is most susceptible. The multi-dose flu vaccine still contains thimerosal. Toxins can cross through the placenta into the fetal bloodstream. So not only are babies in utero being exposed to mercury from adult shots that still contain it, but they are also exposed to aluminum and other metabolic and neurological toxins contained in adult vaccines.

Study title: Thimerosal: clinical, epidemiologic, and biochemical studies[23]; *International Journal of Clinical Chemistry, April 2015*

From the study: "Administration of a single Thimerosal-preserved influenza vaccine during pregnancy resulted in a developing fetus receiving a dose of Hg in excess of the US EPA Hg safety limit from between 1,000,000 times to 10,000 times that safety limit at 1 week of development to 7.6 times to 0.1 times that limit at 38 weeks of development." "Even assuming 99% elimination of the Hg dose by the placenta, a developing fetus even at 16 weeks-old would still receive a dose of Hg greater than 2.5 times the EPA Hg limit for safety." "Given the magnitude in excess of the EPA Hg safety limits presented by exposure to a dose of Thimerosal-preserved vaccine during pregnancy, it is biologically plausible for such exposures to result in fetal/infant death and developmental disability."

Their concluding statement: "The effects of Thimerosal in humans indicates that it is a poison at minute levels with a plethora of deleterious consequences, and there is a clear cause for concern."

Massive amounts of mercury are found in vaccines: The flu vaccine contains 25,000 times more mercury than the EPA allows in drinking water!

In 2014, Natural News publisher Mike Adams, revealed results of the analysis done on the Flulaval flu vaccine. Mercury tests conducted on vaccines at the Natural News Forensic Food Lab have revealed a shockingly high level of toxic mercury in an influenza vaccine (flu shot) made by GlaxoSmithKline (lot #9H2GX). "Tests conducted via ICP-MS document mercury in the Flulaval vaccine at a shocking 51 parts per million, or over 25,000 times higher than the maximum contaminant level of inorganic mercury in drinking water set by the EPA.[86]

In fact, the concentration of mercury found in this GSK flu shot was 100 times higher than the highest level of mercury we've ever tested in contaminated fish. And yet vaccines are injected directly into the body, making them many times more toxic than anything ingested orally."

One question I have is this: How can the EPA tell pregnant mothers not to eat fish more than once per month, for fear that the baby would suffer harm from the mercury, yet the CDC and the FDA promotes injecting much higher amounts of mercury straight into a pregnant woman and consequently into a newborn's blood stream? In answering this question, you also must consider that the fact that absorption of mercury ingested (as in eating fish), is tiny compared to injecting it straight into the blood stream, making the scenario asked in this question more bizarre.

Thimerosal is linked to Reproductive Issues

Study title: A study on the potential reprotoxic effects of thimerosal in male albino rats[87]; *Saudi Journal of Biological Sciences, October 2020*

From the study: "Mercury is one of the most damaging sources of the reproductive system in animals and humans (Boujbiha et al., 2009). By disturbing the thyroid, pituitary, pancreas and adrenal glands, mercury can affect the endocrine systems of humans and animals even at very low concentration (Rice et al., 2014)."

Conclusion of the study: "In conclusion, our findings show that exposure to thimerosal results in increased oxidative stress and decreased activities of antioxidant enzymes, which ultimately lead to impairment in reproductive hormones and eventually decreased daily sperm production in testicular tissues of treated rats".

Mercury from vaccines may cause Premature Puberty

Study title: Thimerosal exposure & increasing trends of premature puberty in the vaccine safety datalink[88], *Indian Journal of Medical Research, April 2010*

Description: Premature puberty is characterized by sexual development before the age of eight in girls, and age 10 in boys. The study looked at 278,624 children born between 1990-1996 and compared the subjects that developed premature puberty to their extent of exposure to Thimerosal Containing Vaccines (TCVs).

From the study: "The overall results of the present study showed a significant association between Hg exposure from thimerosal-containing vaccines and premature puberty. There were significantly increased rate ratios for premature puberty following increasing Hg exposure from thimerosal-containing vaccines administered in the first 7 and 13 months of life."

The study concludes with a discussion of other studies that have shown that mercury disrupts the levels of sex steroid hormones and by binding to receptor sites on ovarian cellular membranes. It also confirmed that many studies have found that mercury has endocrine disrupting effects, and that exposure can lead to hormonal problems.

VACCINES ARE HARMFUL TO THE FETUS DURING PREGNANCY

Influenza vaccine package insert reveals that vaccine recommended for pregnant women has never been tested in pregnant women or children less than 6 months of age for safety or effectiveness

The Influenza A (H1N1) 2009 Monovalent Vaccine manufactured by Sanofi Pasteur Inc. vaccine package insert reveals that: "Safety and effectiveness of influenza A (H1N1) 2009 monovalent vaccine have not been established in pregnant women or nursing mothers or children less than six months of age."[89]

So, they have not established the safety and efficacy of the flu vaccine when given to pregnant women, nursing mothers and children less than six months of age. Despite these shortfalls, CDC still recommends such flu shots for those groups. Yet, the CDC's Advisory Committee was, and is still recommending giving pregnant women these shots.[90]

Even the FDA admits that safety testing was never done on the flu vaccines or the Tdap vaccine in pregnancy, yet both are recommended for pregnant women! Can you believe it?

The CDC recommends that all pregnant women get the flu and Tdap shots. Children's Health Defense recently published an excellent article on this use of untested flu and Tdap vaccines on pregnant women. It reveals that the FDA has no records showing that these vaccines have been safety tested.[91]

Filing a Freedom of Information Act Request, Robert F. Kennedy Jr., on behalf of The Informed Consent Action Network (ICAN) asked the FDA for the following: "A copy of the report for each clinical trial relied upon by the FDA when approving for use by pregnant women any influenza vaccine currently approved by the FDA."

In response, they received the following response from the FDA: "These requests sought the clinical trials relied upon by the FDA prior to approving any currently licensed influenza or Tdap vaccine for use in pregnant women as an indicated use. We have no records responsive to your requests."

So how can our government's committee assigned to oversee the safety and efficacy of vaccines, recommend a vaccine to pregnant women that the manufacturer itself clearly states that there has been no safety and effectiveness studies done with pregnant women or nursing mothers? Doesn't it sound an alarm that these agencies aren't working for welfare of the people?

Miscarriage rates increased by 8x in pregnant women who were given the H1N1 flu shots

Study title: Association of spontaneous abortion with receipt of inactivated influenza vaccine containing H1N1pdm09 in 2010-11 and 2011-12[92]; *Vaccine, September 2017*

Description: The study shows a powerful correlation between pregnant women receiving the H1N1 flu shot and spontaneous abortion (miscarriage) within the next 28 days. It showed a 7.7 times greater risk of miscarriage than the control group.

From the study: "Among women who received pH1N1-containing vaccine in the previous influenza season, the aOR in the 1-28 days was 7.7." (aOR stands for Adjusted Odds Ratio. The Odds Ratio represents the odds that an outcome will occur given a particular exposure, compared to the odds of the outcome occurring in the absence of that exposure). This policy is still being pushed on pregnant mothers to be vaccinated, even though there is no basis science showing the benefit of vaccines in pregnancy.

VACCINES CAUSE ALLERGIES AND ASTHMA CASES

Study title: Is infant immunization a risk factor for childhood asthma or allergy?[93] *Epidemiology, November 1997*

Brief description: This article shows the potential relationship between infant immunization with subsequent development of asthma and allergy. This study was done in New Zealand, and it evaluated a total of 1,265 children. They studied the children who had been vaccinated as an infant with the diphtheria/pertussis/tetanus (DPT) shot and polio.

From the study: "The 23 children who received no diphtheria/pertussis/tetanus (DPT) and polio immunizations had no recorded asthma episodes or consultations for asthma or other allergic illness before age 10 years; in the immunized children, 23.1% had asthma episodes, 22.5% asthma consultations, and 30.0% consultations for other allergic illness. Similar differences were observed at ages 5 and 16 years."

Comments: It shows that none of the unvaccinated children had experienced any asthma or allergy episodes or had any doctor visits. Six years later, they did a follow-up and as of age 16 the results were essentially the same.

From my experience: I have met many vaccine-injured children and their families in my life. I also met a family with 4 children: 3 children took all the childhood vaccines, and 1 child did not take any vaccines. All 3 of the vaccinated children had episodes of asthma, allergies, and eczema whereas the unvaccinated child had none. So, far the unvaccinated child is the healthiest amongst them. It was narrated by the family to me directly.

Another research shows that vaccinated children have 4 times more cases of asthma than unvaccinated children

Study title: Analysis of health outcomes in vaccinated and unvaccinated children: Developmental delays, asthma, ear infections and gastrointestinal disorders[94]; *Sage Open Medicine, May 2020*

From the study: "For asthma the vaccinated group had a 4.49 times (449%) greater prevalence than the unvaccinated group. For development delay the vaccinated group had a 2.18 times (218%) greater prevalence than the unvaccinated group."

VACCINES ARE LINKED TO INSULIN DEPENDENT DIABETES TYPE-1

Vaccination may increase antibodies that can trigger diabetes

Study title: Vaccinations may induce diabetes-related autoantibodies in one-year-old children[95]; *Annals of the New York Academy of Sciences, November 2003*

Description: This paper provides evidence that vaccines contribute to alterations in the immune process that may lead to type 1 diabetes. When analyzing the induction of autoantibodies, the titer levels of IA-2A (sensitive antibody markers associated with the development of type 1 diabetes) were significantly higher in children who received a Hib vaccine.

Thimerosal, aluminum, immunization, and type 1 diabetes

Study title: Prevalence of Autism is Positively Associated with the Incidence of Type 1 Diabetes, but Negatively Associated with the Incidence of Type 2 Diabetes, Implication for the Etiology of the Autism Epidemic[96]; *Open Access Scientific Reports, 2013*

From the study: "Vaccines have shown to cause a large number of cases of type 1 diabetes in both a prospective clinical trial as well as in animal toxicity studies." "The epidemics of type 1 diabetes and autoimmune autism are more likely than not to share the same etiological cause."

Vaccinations increase the risk of diabetes

Study title: Risk of Vaccine Induced Diabetes in Children with a Family History of Type 1 Diabetes[97]; *The Open Pediatric Medicine Journal, 2008*

From the Abstract: "Cohort data from Denmark in all children born from January 1, 1990 to December 31, 2000 was analyzed to assess the association between immunization and type 1 diabetes in all Danish children and in a subgroup where children had a sibling with type 1 diabetes. Pediatric vaccines were associated with a statistically significant increased risk of type 1 diabetes in 12 of 21 endpoints in the general population."

Vaccination linked with insulin-dependent diabetes

Study title: Vaccines and the risk of insulin-dependent diabetes (IDDM): potential mechanism of action[98]; *Medical Hypotheses, November 2001*

From the Abstract: "Immunization with a number of different vaccines, including live and killed vaccines, has been linked to the development of insulin-dependent (type1) diabetes in humans and animals. Multiple different mechanisms have been proposed to explain the association between vaccines and diabetes." "Vaccines are known to manipulate the immune system and can induce an autoimmune disease such as type1 diabetes."

Vaccinations are linked with autoimmune type-1 diabetes and metabolic syndromes like obesity and diabetes type-2

Study title: Review of Vaccine Induced Immune Overload and the Resulting Epidemics of Type 1 Diabetes and Metabolic Syndrome, Emphasis on Explaining the Recent Accelerations in the Risk of Prediabetes and other Immune Mediated Diseases[99]; *Journal of Molecular and Genetic Medicine, 2014*

From the abstract: "Extensive evidence links vaccine induced immune overload with the epidemic of type-1 diabetes. More recent data indicates that obesity, type-2 diabetes, and other components of metabolic syndrome are highly associated with immunization and may be manifestations of the negative feedback loop of the immune system reacting to the immune overload."

"Twenty years ago, it was predicted that a massive increase in immunization would result in a massive increase in people with chronic immune related diseases like type 1 diabetes, autoimmune diseases, and asthma. A massive increase in immunization has occurred. In the United States for example since just 1999 children are scheduled to routinely receive over 80 additional vaccines over their childhood as explained below. The increase in immunization has been followed by a huge increase in inflammation associated disorders. Diseases like autism, type 1 diabetes, asthma, food allergies, many autoimmune diseases, obesity, type 2 diabetes, NASH, and metabolic syndrome have increased many folds in children."

VACCINES INCREASE RISKS OF CNS DISEASES LIKE MULTIPLE SCLEROSIS BY 5X TIMES

2018 study finds up to 5x more chances of developing central nervous demyelinating disease like Multiple Sclerosis in adults given the Hepatitis B vaccine

Study title: Central Demyelinating Diseases after Vaccination Against Hepatitis B Virus: A Disproportionality Analysis within the VAERS Database[100]; *Drug Safety, August 2018*

Method of the study: "We calculated the proportional reporting rate (PRR) and reporting odds ratio (ROR) of MS having occurred within the 120 days following HB immunization in adults aged 19-49 years when compared with other vaccines using the reports recorded in the VAERS database."

Findings from the study: "All computed ratios were found to be statistically significant, with PRRs ranging from 3.48 to 5.56 and RORs ranging from 3.48 to 5.62. When considering the geographical origin, similar RORs were obtained for both US and non-US cases." (That translates into a 350-550% increase in developing central nervous system demyelinating disease like multiple sclerosis).

Conclusion from the study: "In VAERS, MS cases were up to five times more likely to be reported after an HB vaccination than after any other vaccination."

VACCINES ARE SUSPECTED TO CAUSE DNA DAMAGE THAT IS PASSED DOWN MULTIPLE GENERATIONS

Strong evidence suggests that prenatal environmental exposures by chemicals and metals, can cause adult diseases and even generational DNA mutations!

Study title: Prenatal environmental exposures, epigenetics, and disease[101]; *Reproductive Toxicology, April 2011*

Description: It explains how prenatal exposure to toxins including heavy metals and endocrine disrupting chemicals (which are found in numerous vaccines), can lead to DNA mutations and result in disease later in life. The dangerous thing is that these mutations are also thought to carry on to up to 3 or more generations. In other words, if you are exposed to these toxins as a pregnant mother and those toxins create DNA mutations in your child, the same mutations and thus predisposition to resultant disease could be carried down to the woman's grandchildren, great grandchildren, and even great-great grandchildren!

From the article: "This review summarizes recent evidence that prenatal exposure to diverse environmental chemicals dysregulates the fetal epigenome, with potential consequences for subsequent developmental disorders and disease manifesting in childhood, over the life course, or even transgenerationally."

This is of huge importance when it comes to the question of vaccines! Imagine the potential impact of the many chemicals highlighted earlier that are found in vaccines. There are known and suspected carcinogens (causes cancer), mutagens (causes genetic mutations), teratogens (causes malformation of an embryo), endocrine (hormone) disrupting chemicals, heavy metals like mercury and aluminum, neurotoxins, fetotoxins (poisonous to a fetus), neuroexcitatory agents, multiple antibiotics that are not supposed to be given together, solvents, disinfectants, foreign animal and human DNA fragments and retroviruses all found in vaccines! These toxic ingredients have the potential to cause damage to the fetal germ layer developmentally, potentially causing generational defects.

MORE VACCINE DOSES IMPLIES MORE CASES OF SPEECH AND LANGUAGE DISORDERS

Number of vaccine doses correlates with rates of autism and speech and language impairment in the U.S.

Study title: A positive association found between autism prevalence and childhood vaccination uptake across the U.S. population[102]; *Journal of Toxicology and Environmental Health, 2011*

From the abstract: "A positive and statistically significant relationship was found: The higher the proportion of children receiving recommended vaccinations, the higher was the prevalence of autism (AUT) or speech or language impairment (SLI). A 1% increase in vaccination was associated with an additional 680 children having AUT or SLI."

VACCINES AND CHILDHOOD OBESITY: A STRONG CONNECTION

Study title: Thimerosal-containing Hepatitis B Vaccine Exposure is Highly Associated with Childhood Obesity: A Case-control Study Using the Vaccine Safety Datalink[103]; *North American Journal of Medical Sciences, July 2016*

Conclusions: "In a dose-response manner, the present study associates an increased organic mercury exposure from Thimerosal-containing hepatitis B vaccines with an increased risk of obesity diagnosis and suggests that Thimerosal is an obesogen." (Causes obesity)

VACCINES CAN TRIGGER AUTO-IMMUNE DISEASES LIKE RHEAUMATOID ARTHRITIS

Vaccine association with Rheumatoid Arthritis (RA)

Study title: Joint and limb symptoms in children after immunisation with measles, mumps, and rubella vaccine[104]; *British Medical Journal, April 1992*

Description: The study evaluated the incidence of joint manifestations within 6 weeks after MMR immunization: it included 2658 vaccinated and 2359 non-vaccinated children, confirming an increased risk of joint symptoms (arthralgia or arthritis) in the immunized children.

Conclusions from the study: "Measles, mumps, and rubella vaccine is associated with an increased risk of episodes of joint and limb symptoms, especially in girls and children under 5. The risk of frank arthritis is substantially less than after wild rubella infection."

Vaccinations can trigger the paralytic autoimmune syndrome called Guillain-Barré syndrome

Study title: Clinical Features of Post-Vaccination Guillain-Barré Syndrome (GBS) in Korea[105]; *Journal of Korean Medical Science, July 2017*

Description: GBS is the most common immune-mediated polyradiculoneuropathy and it is also the most commonly reported severe adverse event following immunization in adults according to the study.

From the study: "G.B.S. is an acute or subacute peripheral polyneuropathy, which is accompanied by symmetric flaccid paralysis of the extremities, sensory abnormalities, and cranial nerve palsy."

"Interest in the risk of GBS after vaccination increased after approximately 500 cases of GBS were reported after the mass administration of the A/New Jersey/76 vaccine during the swine flu epidemic in the United States in 1976." "In addition to influenza vaccines, cases of GBS have been reported after immunization with various vaccines, including measles, mumps, and rubella (MMR), hepatitis B, diphtheria, tetanus, and pertussis (DTP) and polio."

VACCINES CAN CAUSE INFLAMMATION OF THE HEART (MYOCARDITIS/PERICARDITIS)

Flu Shot may lead to Pericarditis, i.e., Inflammation of the covering of the heart - a serious cardiovascular issue

Study title: Pericarditis. Series of 84 consecutive cases[106]; *Arquivos Brasileiros de Cardiologia, April 2004*

Description: This study found a very strong association between the flu shot and cases of pericarditis in individuals that had not been previously diagnosed.

Method of the study: From January 1999 to December 2001, 84 patients with clinically and echocardiographically diagnosed pericarditis were identified in a heart clinic. The individuals were divided into 2 groups: group A comprised 61 patients with known causes of pericarditis and group B comprised 23 patients with idiopathic (unknown) causes.

Results from the study: "Twenty-three (100%) group B patients received anti-influenza vaccine versus none in group A."

THE TRUTH OF FLU SHOT: ZERO BENEFIT WITH IMMENSE RISK

Influenza Vaccines may increase the risk of Influenza

Study title: Association between the 2008—09 seasonal influenza vaccine and pandemic HINI illness during Spring— summer 2009: four observational studies from Canada[107]; *PLoS Medicine, April 2010*

Description: Four studies showed that recipients of a seasonal influenza vaccine had a significantly increased risk of subsequently developing severe pandemic influenza (H1N1) compared to people who did not receive the seasonal vaccine.

Children who got the flu shot had no reduction in flu cases but higher rate of other respiratory illness within 14 days

Study title: Assessment of temporally-related acute respiratory illness following influenza vaccination[108]; *Vaccine, April 2018*

Description: The study found that children who are vaccinated for influenza develop a higher rate of non-influenza acute respiratory illness in the 14 days after the vaccination than those that are not vaccinated.

Results from the study: "The hazard of influenza in individuals during the 14-day post-vaccination period was similar to unvaccinated individuals during the same period."

Conclusion of the study: "Among children there was an increase in the hazard of ARI (Acute Respiratory Illness) caused by non-influenza respiratory pathogens post-influenza vaccination compared to unvaccinated children during the same period."

The influenza vaccine may increase the risk of other respiratory infections by 4 times

Study title: Increased Risk of Non-influenza Respiratory Virus Infections Associated with Receipt of Inactivated Influenza Vaccine[109]; *Clinical Infectious Diseases, June 2012*

Description: The study challenges the thinking that immunization against the flu reduces flu symptoms such as upper respiratory infections. The reality is that vaccination against the flu appears to increase the rates of other non-influenza upper respiratory infections by greater than 400%!

From the study: "We randomized 115 children to trivalent inactivated influenza vaccine (TIV) or placebo. Over the following 9 months, IV recipients had an increased risk of virologically confirmed non-influenza infections." "TIV recipients may lack temporary non-specific immunity that protected against other respiratory viruses."

Mainstream pediatric journal finds the influenza vaccine completely ineffective in children under five years of age

Study title: Influenza vaccine effectiveness among children 6 to 59 months of age during 2 influenza seasons: a case-cohort study[110]; *Archives of Pediatrics and Adolescent Medicine, October 2008*

Conclusion of the study: "In 2 seasons with suboptimal antigenic match between vaccines and circulating strains, we could not demonstrate VE (Vaccine effectiveness) in preventing influenza-related inpatient/ED or outpatient visits in children younger than 5 years."

Children that get the influenza vaccine have 3 times the risk of subsequent hospitalization, as documented by researchers at the Mayo Clinic

Report title: Flu Vaccination May Triple Risk for Flu-Related Hospitalization in Children with Asthma[111]; *American Thoracic Society, May 2009*

Description: The report looked at children over a 10-year period who did and did not receive the flu vaccine. It was determined that children that got the flu vaccine were 3 times more likely to be hospitalized than those that were not vaccinated.

From the report: "In order to determine whether the vaccine was effective in reducing the number of hospitalizations that all children, and especially the ones with asthma, faced over eight consecutive flu seasons, the researchers conducted a cohort study of 263 children who were evaluated at the Mayo Clinic in Minnesota from six months to 18 years of age, each of whom had had laboratory-confirmed influenza between 1996 to 2006. The investigators determined who had and had not received the flu vaccine, their asthma status and who did and did not require hospitalization. Records were reviewed for each subject with influenza-related illness for flu vaccination preceding the illness and hospitalization during that illness.

"They found that children who had received the flu vaccine had three times the risk of hospitalization, as compared to children who had not received the vaccine. In asthmatic children, there was a significantly higher risk of hospitalization in subjects who received the Trivalent Influenza Vaccine, as compared to those who did not (p= 0.006)."

A 2018 Cochrane Review of 52 studies on the effectiveness of the flu vaccine in over 80,000 healthy adults shows that being vaccinated maybe only 1% better than not being vaccinated

Study title: Vaccines for preventing influenza in healthy adults[112]; *The Cochrane Database of Systematic Reviews, February 2018.*

From the study: "Healthy adults who receive inactivated parenteral influenza vaccine rather than no vaccine probably experience less influenza, from just over 2% to just under 1% (moderate-certainty evidence)." "71 healthy adults need to be vaccinated to prevent one of them experiencing influenza."

Fifteen included trials were industry funded (29%). This is interesting. What I mean by that is, if nearly a third of the studies they looked at were funded by the drug industry (and you can bet they put their best numbers forward), and that didn't even skew the results in their favor, most likely the non-drug industry studies found even less or no benefit at all.

So, one must ask himself, is it worth playing Russian Roulette with all the toxic ingredients from the flu vaccine to have negligible benefit at all? Why not just optimize the vitamin and mineral levels, eat healthy, get quality sleep, practice good hygiene and we could lower the risk much more than risking the flu shot. 72 hours water fasting, or juice fasting has enormously great results as were seen by Network of Influenza Care Experts who cured more than 60,000 patients of Covid-19 symptoms in 2020-21. I was a member of the network and cared for more than 250 patients.

MEASLES, MUMPS AND RUBBELA (MMR) VACCINE: ONE OF THE MOST DANGEROUS VACCINES

The MMR Cover-up and Scandal

Former Chief Scientific Officer fears the MMR vaccine causes serious risk of brain damage and implicates a cover-up by "powerful" people

This article from The Daily Mail, titled Former science chief: 'MMR fears coming true'[113] features Dr. Peter Fletcher, the former Chief Scientific Officer at the Department of Health in Great Britain. Dr. Fletcher also served as the Medical Assessor to the Committee on Safety of Medicines, meaning he was responsible for deciding if new vaccines were safe.

He has seen a "steady accumulation of evidence" from scientists worldwide that the measles, mumps, and rubella jab is causing brain damage in certain children. But he added: "There are very powerful people in positions of great authority in Britain and elsewhere who have staked their reputations and careers on the safety of MMR, and they are willing to do almost anything to protect themselves."

The Bombshell Revelation: The scientists at the CDC falsified data on the MMR trials to cover up an association between the MMR vaccine and autism.

Dr. Thompson was a senior scientist and researcher with the CDC and involved with Dr. Frank DeStefano, as co-authors of the now infamous study by the CDC seemingly "proving" a lack of connection between the MMR vaccine and autism. The 2004 study was titled, MMR vaccine and autism: an update of the scientific evidence and published in Expert Review of Vaccines. This seminal study attempting to finally put the question about the connection between autism and the MMR shot to rest, has been rocked by allegations from Dr. Thompson that he and the researchers had "cooked the books".

To Dr. Thompson's credit, after 13 years his conscience finally got the best of him. Dr. Thompson has admitted that the researchers had changed criteria and the methods of the study to skew the results. He said they also collaborated to destroy documents to hide the evidence, which showed when the MMR shots were given to African American boys before 36 months of age, they had a 250% greater risk of developing autism. According to Dr. Thompson, in 2002 they brought in large trash cans and required all the researchers to bring the data they were holding showing the association with the increase in autism and throw them into the cans for destruction.

Fortunately, Dr. Thompson felt uneasy about the fraud and kept copies of the original documents, which he has turned over to Brian Hooker, an investigative reporter. The following is from an article about Dr. Thompson and his revelations published on the web site of an organization named 'A Voice for Choice'. Their mission statement states: A Voice for Choice promotes people's rights to make fully informed choices and know the composition, quality and short and long-term health effects of food and pharmaceutical products.

Dr. William Thompson stated: "I regret that my coauthors and I omitted statistically significant information in our 2004 article published in the journal Pediatrics. The omitted data suggested that African American males who received the MMR vaccine before age 36 months were at increased risk for autism. "[114]

"My concern has been the decision to omit relevant findings in a particular study for a particular subgroup for a particular vaccine. There have always been recognized risks for vaccination and I believe it is the responsibility of the CDC to properly convey the risks associated with receipt of those vaccines."

Dr. William Thompson is an author of two of the three epidemiological studies touted by the CDC to prove the safety of Thimerosal. He is also coauthor of the CDC's 2004 DeStefano study which dismissed the link between the MMR vaccine and autism. It is cited by the CDC and vaccine industry to claim that vaccines do not cause autism. Dr. Thompson now confesses that he and his fellow CDC researchers found a strong autism signal in children who received the MMR vaccine before their third birthday. According to him, the scientists eliminated this data from the final published study under orders from their bosses.

Comments: The CDC claims to be an 'independent' watchdog, but by definition, it is a private corporation working on behalf of its stakeholders, which include key players in the pharmaceutical and vaccine industries that profit from the spread of disease, not from real prevention and cures.

Did the Measles Vaccine Eradicate Measles? No!

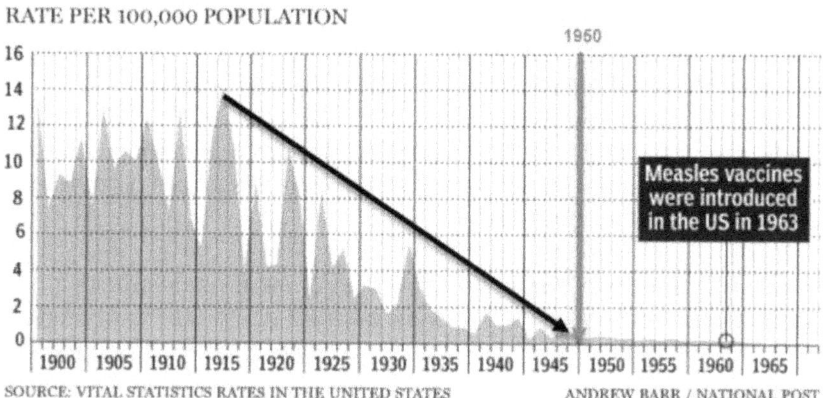

In the above graph, you can see the steep decline of measles deaths throughout the 20th Century, with the steep downward trajectory from its peak in 1915 to 1963 when the measles vaccine was introduced. For the pharmaceutical industry and medical doctors to claim that vaccines save thousands of deaths annually is simply a lie. How can vaccines get the credit for around 99% reduction in deaths before the vaccine even existed?[115] [116] [117]

There was a sharp decline of the measles disease attributed to better nutrition, sanitation, access to clean water, waste disposal, public health measures, personal hygiene education, etc. not the vaccine. In other words, if the measles vaccine was never used, the rate of deaths due to measles would still be right where we are today.

Injuries and deaths from the Measles (MMR) Vaccine

Article title: Measles Disease & Vaccine Information[118]; *National Vaccine Information Centre*

From the article: "As of May 31, 2019, there have been more than 94,972 reports of measles-vaccine reactions, hospitalizations, injuries, and deaths following measles vaccinations made to the federal Vaccine Adverse Events Reporting System, including 468 related deaths, 7,127 hospitalizations, and 1,820 related disabilities. Over 50% of those adverse events occurred in children three years old and under."

Measles outbreak happened in vaccinated students

The historical reality that no one seems to ever mention in the media, is that according to US Vital Statistics reports over the course of the 20th century, measles deaths had declined by around 99% before the vaccine was ever introduced. But we all know if we listen to media reports, vaccines get all the credit. But do the vaccines even work?

Study title: Failure to reach the goal of measles elimination. Apparent paradox of measles infections in immunized persons[119]; *Archives of Internal Medicine, August 1994*

Results of the study: "We found 18 reports of measles outbreaks in very highly immunized school populations where 71% to 99.8% of students were immunized against measles. Despite these high rates of immunization, 30% to 100% (mean, 77%) of all measles cases in these outbreaks occurred in previously immunized students."

Conclusions of the study: "The apparent paradox is that as measles immunization rates rise to high levels in a population, measles becomes a disease of immunized persons. Because of the failure rate of the vaccine and the unique transmissibility of the measles virus, the currently available measles vaccine, used in a single-dose strategy, is unlikely to completely eliminate measles."

130% more cases of measles were found in the population that got more doses of the measles vaccine

Study title: Largest measles epidemic in North America in a decade--Quebec, Canada, 2011: contribution of susceptibility, serendipity, and superspreading events[120]; *Journal of Infectious Diseases, March 2013*

Results from the study: "There were 21 measles importations and 725 cases. A superspreading event triggered by 1 importation resulted in sustained transmission and 678 cases. The overall incidence was 9.1 per 100,000; the highest incidence was in adolescents 12-17 years old (75.6 per 100,000), who comprised 56% of case patients. Among adolescents, 22% had received 2 vaccine doses. Outbreak investigation showed this proportion to have been an underestimate; active case finding identified 130% more cases among 2-dose recipients."

HPV VACCINE IS HIGHLY TOXIC: DOES NOT PREVENT CERVICAL CANCER

HPV Vaccine causes disability and deaths

As of December 2019, "VAERS has logged 64270 adverse reactions related to the HPV vaccine. Among those, 3092 are listed as "disabled," 13072 are listed as "did not recover," 9497 are listed as "serious," and 523 deaths have been reported. Many other reports of side effects were posted in VAERS which are shown in the table below.[121]

EVENTS REPORTED TO VAERS AFTER HPV VACCINES THROUGH DEC 14, 2019

Event	Female	Male	Unknown	Totals
Disabled	2869	141	82	3092
Deaths	392	31	100	523
Did Not Recover	11,801	996	275	13,072
Abnormal Smear	688	1	6	695
Cervical Cancer	180	0	6	186
Infertility	52	1	0	53
Life Threatening	897	88	16	1,001
Emergency Room	13,664	1,581	174	15,419
Hospitalization	5,956	379	113	6,448
Extended Hospital Stay	285	18	1	304
Serious	8,692	529	276	9,497
TOTAL REPORTS	45,235	7,599	11,436	64,270

HPV Vaccine is responsible for the third highest number of vaccine court compensation awards at 126 through 2016. The DTaP vaccine and its versions is second (208 through 2016) and the flu vaccine is responsible for the highest number of vaccine court compensation awards (2,439 through 2016).[122]

No evidence proves that HPV vaccination can prevent cervical cancer; However, serious adverse reactions are common!

Study title: Human papillomavirus (HPV) vaccine policy and evidence-based Medicine: are they at odds?[123] *Annals of Medicine, March 2013*

From the study: "While the world's leading medical authorities state that HPV vaccines are an important cervical cancer prevention tool, clinical trials show no evidence that HPV vaccination can protect against cervical cancer." "Cumulatively, the list of serious adverse reactions related to HPV vaccination worldwide includes deaths, convulsions, paraesthesia, paralysis, Guillain–Barré syndrome (GBS), transverse myelitis, facial palsy, chronic fatigue syndrome, anaphylaxis, autoimmune disorders, deep vein thrombosis, pulmonary embolisms, and cervical cancers."

Ten percent of women taking HPV vaccine had an emergency room visit or were hospitalized in the following 42 days

Study title: Adverse events following HPV vaccination, Alberta 2006–2014[124]; *Vaccine, April 2016*

Results of the study: "Over the period 195,270 females received 528,913 doses of HPV vaccine." "Of the women who received HPV vaccine 958 were hospitalized and 19,351 (10%) had an ED visit within 42 days of immunization."

HPV vaccine may lower a woman's chance of getting pregnant It is associated with Premature Ovarian Insufficiency (Infertility – Early menopause)

Study title: A lowered probability of pregnancy in females in the USA aged 25-29 who received a human papillomavirus vaccine injection[125]; *Journal of Toxicology and Environmental Health, 2018*

Description: This study finds that a disproportionate percentage of women that have had the HPV vaccine have been unable to conceive versus the women that have never had the shot. The HPV Vaccine has been associated with a condition called Premature Ovarian Insufficiency making them infertile, which is essentially early menopause.

From the Abstract: "Birth rates in the United States have recently fallen. Birth rates per 1000 females aged 25-29 fell from 118 in 2007 to 105 in 2015. One factor may involve the vaccination against the human papillomavirus (HPV). Shortly after the vaccine was licensed, several reports of recipients experiencing primary ovarian failure emerged. This study analyzed information gathered in National Health and Nutrition Examination Survey, which represented 8 million 25-to-29-year-old women residing in the United States between 2007 and 2014.

Results: "Approximately 60% of women who did not receive the HPV vaccine had been pregnant at least once, whereas only 35% of women who were exposed to the vaccine had conceived. For married women, 75% who did not receive the shot were found to conceive, while only 50% who received the vaccine had ever been pregnant. Using logistic regression to analyze the data, the probability of having been pregnant was estimated for females who received an HPV vaccine compared with females who did not receive the shot.

"Results suggest that females who received the HPV shot were less likely to have ever been pregnant than women in the same age group who did not receive the shot. If 100% of females in this study had received the HPV vaccine, data suggest the number of women having ever conceived would have fallen by 2 million. Further study into the influence of HPV vaccine on fertility is thus warranted."

Twenty-one-year-old woman's death was finally compensated in 2017 after eight years, as the court rules that the HPV vaccine caused her death

Natural News reported on a case whereby a 21-year-old woman (Christina Richelle), developed an irregular heartbeat, days after receiving her second HPV vaccine Gardasil in November of 2007. Within days after she returned for her third HPV dose in June of 2008. For several days after that third shot, she felt dizzy. Her heart malfunctioned and she died later.

It was determined that she had developed an autoimmune reaction that affected the electrical system of her heart. The family filed a petition to the vaccine court in April 2010. After nearly eight years of battling the court process, the court ruled that the family provided sufficient medical burden of proof that Christina's death was attributed to the Gardasil vaccine, and they were due for compensation under the Vaccine Injury Protection Act.[126]

DIPTHERIA, TETANUS, PERTUSSIS VACCINE (DTaP) IS HIGHLY POISONOUS AND INEFFECTIVE

New evidence that the DPT Vaccine in Africa kills more children from other causes than it saves from Diphtheria, Pertussis, or Tetanus

Study title: The Introduction of Diphtheria-Tetanus-Pertussis and Oral Polio Vaccine Among Young Infants in an Urban African Community: A Natural Experiment[127]; *E BioMedicine, March 2017*

Description: The lead author is famous for his work with vaccines in third world countries. He decided to look back at the data from the early 1980's and what he found was very alarming. Children that got the DPT vaccine had a 5x greater mortality (death) than those that did not get it. They did not die from diphtheria, pertussis, or tetanus. They died from seizures, and other kinds of infections. Their immune systems were compromised by the DPT vaccine.

From the article: "DTP was associated with 5-fold higher mortality than being unvaccinated. No prospective study has shown beneficial survival effects of DTP." "All currently available evidence suggests that DTP vaccine may kill more children from other causes than it saves from diphtheria, tetanus or pertussis."

DTP vaccine increases the cases of allergies and asthma

Study title: Effects of diphtheria-tetanus-pertussis or tetanus vaccination on allergies and allergy-related respiratory symptoms among children and adolescents in the United States[128]; *Journal of Manipulative and Physiological Therapeutics, February 2000*

Results: "The odds of having a history of asthma was twice as great among vaccinated subjects than among unvaccinated subjects (adjusted odds ratio, 2.00)." "The odds of having had any allergy-related respiratory symptom in the past 12 months was 63% greater among vaccinated subjects than unvaccinated subjects (adjusted odds ratio 1.63)."

Conclusions from the study: "DTP or tetanus vaccination appears to increase the risk of allergies and related respiratory symptoms in children and adolescents."

The DPT vaccine causes high rates of severe adverse reactions: The Pertussis component of DPT was the worst!

Study title: Nature and rates of adverse reactions associated with DTP and DT immunizations in infants and children[129]; *Pediatrics, 1981*

Description: The study compared the adverse reactions between the DTP and the DT (without the Pertussis component) vaccines. It really is a glaring piece of evidence that shows that the Pertussis component was responsible for many adverse reactions from DPT. Bear in mind that these were only reactions that occurred within 48 hours. Many of the reactions including very severe ones from DPT occurred beyond the first 48 hours.

The Abstract: "In 784 DT and 15,752 DTP immunizations given to children 0 to 6 years of age who were prospectively studied for reactions occurring within 48 hours following immunization, minor reactions were significantly more frequent following DTP vaccine."

"The ratio of reaction rates associated with DTP and DT immunizations (DTP/DT) for selected local and systemic reactions was as follows: local redness, 37.4%/7.6%; local swelling, 40.7%/7.6%; pain, 50.9%/9.9%; fever, 31.5%/14.9%; drowsiness, 31.5%/14.9%; fretfulness, 53.4%/22.6%; vomiting, 6.2%/2.6%; anorexia, 20.9%/7.0% and persistent crying, 3.1%/0.7%. Following DTP immunization nine children developed convulsions and nine developed hypotonic hyporesponsive episodes. No sequelae were detected following these reactions."

Tetanus vaccine is highly ineffective

Report title: Tetanus Surveillance --- United States, 2001—2008[130]; *Morbidity and Mortality Weekly Report CDC, April 2011*

The report states that between the years 2001-2008, there were 233 cases of tetanus in the U.S. That works out to an average of 33 per year or about 1 case per 10 million people.

Of those 233 cases over the 7 years, vaccination status was known for 92 of those individuals. Of those 92, 55 (59.3%), had been previously vaccinated. Of the 55 that had been previously vaccinated, 26 had received one dose, 5 had received 3 doses, 24 had received equal to or greater than 4 doses. In addition, medical histories were known for 195 of the cases. Of those 195, 30 reported to have diabetes, 27 were injectable drug users.

That being the case, of the 195 cases discussed 57 (29%), were in individuals with serious pre-existing health and risk factor issues. An important point to take away from this is, that the 138 (71%), remaining "healthy or healthier" people that don't have those 2 serious health risk factors reduce the overall annual incidence of tetanus from 33 per year to just over 23 (23.4%) cases in the U.S.

Therefore, the incidence in those without diabetes or injectable drug users is approximately 1 in 14 million. Considering that there are numerous other health conditions that predispose people to infection, I would submit that the rate of tetanus in truly healthy people is far less than 1 in 14 million.

From the report: "During 2001–2008, the average annual incidence of tetanus in the United States was 0.10 cases overall per 1 million population and 0.23 among persons aged ≥65 years; the case-fatality rate was 13.2% overall but 31.3% among persons aged ≥65 years." The article states that one of the reasons for the precipitous decline in the incidence of tetanus in the U.S. is better wound care.

Comment: To give perspective to the fatality of the disease, the chance of getting struck by lightning is approximately 1 in 700,000, you are 20 times more likely to be struck by lightning in any given year than you are to become infected with tetanus.[131]

A whooping cough outbreak despite high immunization rates proves the pertussis vaccine to be ineffective

Report title: Immunized People Getting Whooping Cough[132]; *KPBS San Diego June 2014*

Description: This report revealed that 85% (527) of the 621 people that contracted whooping cough in San Diego County were up to date on their immunizations against the disease. The investigation led to several scientific studies which found that immunity faded sooner than expected after people were vaccinated.

TRUTH OF HEPATITIS B VACCINE: MAY MULTIPLY THE RISK OF AUTISM

Hepatitis B Vaccine in the first month of life, increases the risk of Autism in boys by 300%

Study title: Hepatitis B vaccination of male neonates and autism diagnosis, NHIS 1997-2002[133]; *Journal of Toxicology and Environmental Health, 2010*

From the abstract: "This cross-sectional study used weighted probability samples obtained from National Health Interview Survey 1997-2002 data sets. Vaccination status was determined from the vaccination record."

"Boys vaccinated as neonates had threefold greater odds for autism diagnosis compared to boys never vaccinated or vaccinated after the first month of life."

"Findings suggest that U.S. male neonates vaccinated with the hepatitis B vaccine prior to 1999 (from vaccination record) had a threefold higher risk for parental report of autism diagnosis compared to boys not vaccinated as neonates during that same time period."

THE TRUTH OF CHICKENPOX VACCINE: INEFFECTIVE AND HARMFUL

The Varicella (Chickenpox) Vaccine - Ineffective and poses other health risks

Study title: Vaccination to prevent varicella: Goldman and King's response to Myers' interpretation of Varicella Active Surveillance Project data[134]; *Human and Experimental Toxicology, 2014*

Description: This study states that not only is the chickenpox vaccine ineffective and inefficient, it also has contributed to the dramatic rise in adult shingles cases.

From the study: "When the costs of the booster dose for varicella and the increased shingles recurrences are included, the universal varicella vaccination program is neither effective nor cost-effective."

The benefit of the Chickenpox vaccine is short lived and increases the risk of hospitalization (by 10-15 times) and death (by 20 times) in older people

Study title: Review of the United States universal varicella vaccination program: Herpes zoster incidence rates, cost-effectiveness, and vaccine efficacy based primarily on the Antelope Valley Varicella Active Surveillance Project data[135]; *Vaccine 2013*

Description: The study cites the usually benign naturally acquired chickenpox providing long-tern immunity as superior to the temporary immunity of the vaccine variety, which they say has compromised the protection of the population afforded by the natural immunity. The authors claim this shifts the disease to an older population, which increases the risk of death by 20 times and hospitalization by 10-15 times.

Conclusion: "Prior to the universal varicella vaccination program, 95% of adults experienced natural chickenpox (usually as pre-school to early elementary school children)—these cases were usually benign. In the prelicensure (vaccine) era, the periodic exogenous boosting that adults received from those shedding VZV resulted in long-term immunity.

(Meaning that adults who had previously contracted chicken pox were exposed to children with it, it would boost their natural immunity)."

"This high percentage of seropositive individuals and their long-term immunity have been compromised by the universal varicella vaccination of children which provides at best 70–90% protection that is temporary and of unknown duration—shifting chickenpox to a more vulnerable adult population which, as Dr. Jane Seward cautioned in 2007, carries 20 times more risk of death and 10–15 times more risk of hospitalization compared to chickenpox in children."

"Thus, the proponents for universal varicella vaccination have failed to consider increased HZ-related morbidity as well as the adverse effects of both the varicella and HZ vaccines which have more than offset the limited benefits associated with reductions in varicella disease."

The universal varicella (chickenpox) vaccination program now requires a booster vaccine for children and an HZ vaccine to boost protection in adults. However, these are less effective than the natural immunity that existed in communities prior to licensure of the varicella vaccine. Hence, rather than eliminating varicella in children as promised, routine vaccination against varicella has proven extremely costly and has created continual cycles of treatment and disease."

THE TRUTH OF SHINGLES VACCINE: INEFFECTIVE AND HARMFUL

Zostavax shingles vaccine is found to be ineffective, and it may cause shingles, vision loss, and many other side effects

Article title: Merck Admits Shingles Vaccine Can Cause Eye Damage and Shingles[136]; *The Children's Medical Safety Research Institute, October 2016*

From the article: "Two important FDA approved changes to the warning label of Merck Pharmaceutical's shingles vaccine, Zostavax, have been made since the controversial drug was introduced in 2006. The first was in August 2014, when, in addition to potentially causing chickenpox, another side effect was added: shingles! That's right. The vaccine that had been – and continues to be -- aggressively marketed to prevent seniors from contracting this excruciating condition was found to actually cause shingles in some individuals."

"In February of this year, the FDA approved a label change to warn those who prescribe the Zostavax vaccine of another potential side effect: "Eye Disorders: necrotizing retinitis." "This disorder, as well as keratitis, causes inflammation and scarring of the eye tissue and can lead to permanent vision loss if not treated quickly. It was reported by WebMD 20 individuals (children and adults) developed keratitis within a month of receiving a chickenpox or shingles vaccine. Keratitis symptoms for adults developed within 24 days of vaccination, while symptoms in children began within14 days of vaccination."

"According to the authors of a Health Sciences Institute (HSI) article in January 2016, "UCLA researchers found that only one in 175 people who get the vaccine will be able to dodge a shingles flare-up." While Merck claims Zostavax is 50% effective, in the placebo group, 3.3 percent of the study participants developed shingles, compared to 1.6 percent in the vaccine group. So, while that is a 50% difference, the real, absolute risk reduction is just 1.7 percentage points."

SMALLPOX VACCINE CAN CAUSE RARE DISEASES AND SEVERAL HEALTH COMPLICATIONS

The smallpox vaccine carries a risk of deadly encephalitis

Study title: The smallpox vaccine and postvaccinal encephalitis[137]; *Seminars in Neurology, March 2002*

From the Abstract: "There were, however, complications associated with smallpox vaccination; the most serious complication was postvaccinal encephalitis, which was reported to occur with an incidence of 1 in 110,000 vaccinations and a case-fatality rate of 50%."

Smallpox vaccine has the strongest association with Myocarditis (Inflammation of Heart) according to a study

Study title: Myocarditis secondary to smallpox vaccination[42]; *British Medical Journal Case Reports, March 2018*

From the Abstract: "Although myocarditis has been reported following many different vaccines, the smallpox vaccine has the strongest association. We report a case of a 36-year-old active-duty service member presenting with progressive dyspnoea, substernal chest pain and lower extremity swelling 5 weeks after receiving the vaccinia vaccination. The aetiology of his acute decompensated heart failure was determined to be from myocarditis. Although the majority of cases of myocarditis resolve completely, some patients develop chronic heart failure and even death. Vaccine-associated myocarditis should always be on the differential for patients that exhibit cardiopulmonary symptoms after recent vaccinations."

TRUTH OF POLIO VACCINE: MAY CAUSE PARALYSIS

Is polio (paralysis) eradicated? No!
Did polio vaccine eradicate it? No!

Article title: CDC and Friends Sprinting Towards the Polio "Finish Line,"[138]; *Suzanne Humphries MD, June 2012*

Many believe that a disease called "polio" has been eradicated in the Western hemisphere. Most everyone thinks that "polio" was eradicated by vaccination. To fully understand where polio went, one must understand what polio was. When one understands what polio was, it becomes clear that it is impossible to eradicate it with a vaccine. But that never stops vaccination interests from launching full- scale propaganda misinformation campaigns in order to vaccinate the children of the world, even though they fail in eliminating paralysis. "Wild" poliovirus may be gone from vaccinated countries, but what was once called "polio," and frightened the wits out of parents world-wide, is still ubiquitous.

The term "poliomyelitis" is a description of spinal pathology. The meaning of the word comes from Greek: polios = gray, and muelos = marrow, it is = inflammation; meaning "inflammation of the gray matter of the spinal cord." All poliomyelitis means is that the gray matter of the spinal cord is inflamed. This can occur anywhere from the brainstem to the end of the spinal cord, and it has always had many causes, the least of which is a virus that lives in intestines of healthy people. The result of this inflammation, whether chemical or viral, leads to certain characteristic muscular symptoms that have been conditioned into the minds of several generations of people to appear as the classic atrophied limbs, iron lungs and other horrifying images.

By definition and by historical documentation, these infamous images of polio should by no means be blamed solely on a specific wild-type (naturally occurring) virus. Environmental toxins, other infections, and laboratory-derived vaccine viruses were all implicated in paralytic polio over the years. Yet wild virus, even though it is said to be asymptomatic in 95% of infected, and only causes paralysis in a small amount of infected is the excuse for world-wide polio vaccination with live viruses that are known to cause their own outbreaks of polio in China, Nigeria, and India. The only difference is that the name of the paralysis has been changed (i.e., Acute Flaccid Paralysis which can be caused by numerous viral and chemical agents, including DDT) and it in many cases is being caused by the polio vaccines themselves.

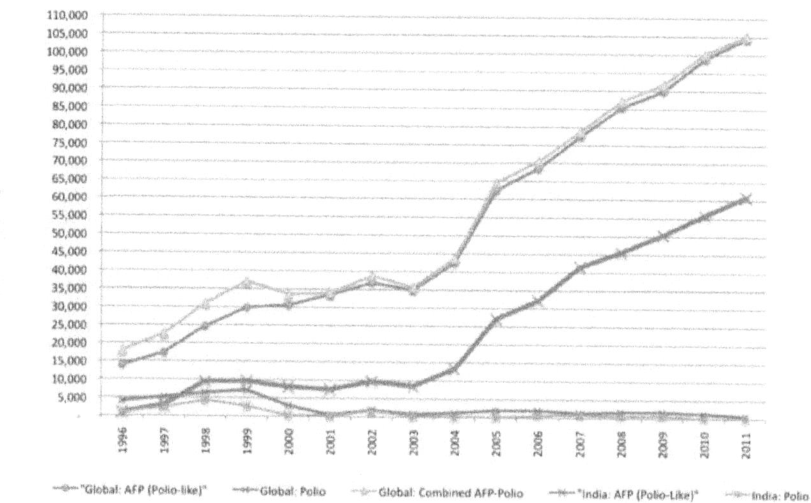

What can we understand from the graph? We can see that the cases of polio (paralysis) are declining but the cases of acute flaccid paralysis are increasing. Which means, the paralysis problem is still there, and it has been increasing with the increase in polio vaccine compliance. Polio was declared to be eradicated but that is a false alarm, the polio "vaccine" paralyzes thousands of children in India even today along with other toxic chemicals consumed by Indian manufacturing industry.

Polio Disease and its association with chemicals like DDT, BHC, Lead and Arsenic

Article title: Pesticides and Polio: A Critique of Scientific Literature[139]; *Jim West, February 2003*

This excellent article details the use of these chemicals and the incredible correlation with the rise and fall of polio prior to the vaccine's introduction is astounding! The use of these chemicals was rampant and their toxic effects on humans was denied for decades. The article even shows dairy farmers spraying DDT on dairy cows in a barn. All the above-mentioned chemicals lead to neurological damage and polio like symptoms. And, since the diagnosis of polio back then was based on a symptomatic presentation and typically did not involve laboratory confirmation, it would've been easy to mis-identify this poisoning for the polio virus.

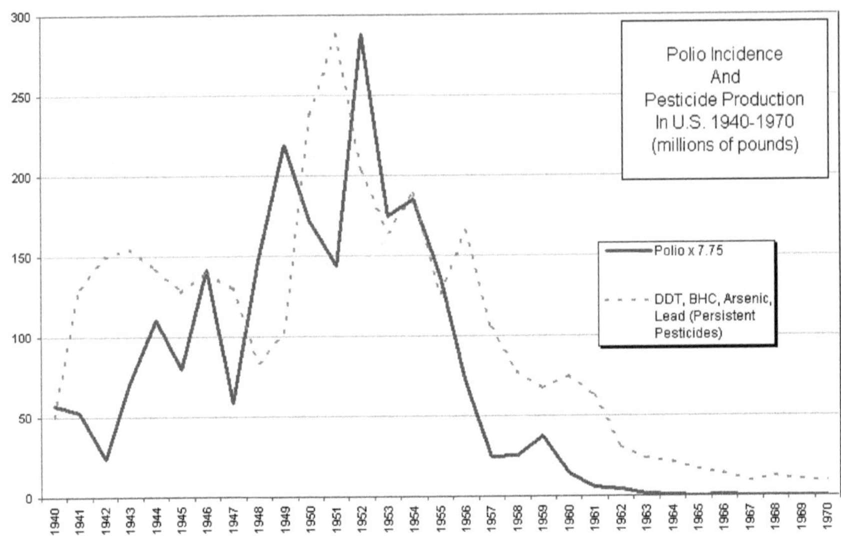

What can we understand from the above graph? We can see that when the use of chemicals like DDT, BHC, Arsenic, lead increased, the cases of polio (paralysis) also increased and vice-versa. It indicates that polio cases (paralysis) are related to chemical toxicity more than the virus.

Polio vaccine might cause Acute Flaccid Paralysis (AFP)

Study title: Polio programme: let us declare victory and move on[140]; *Indian Journal of Medical Ethics, April-June 2012*

Description: The study describes an epidemic of what is called non-polio acute flaccid paralysis (NPAFP), that correlates directly with the use of the oral polio vaccine. There were 47,500 cases occurring in 2011 alone! While affluent countries have moved on to "safer" inactivated forms of the polio vaccine, children in many third world countries have been subjected to using the left-over stock of the live oral version.

From the abstract: "It was hoped that following polio eradication, immunisation could be stopped. However, the synthesis of polio virus in 2002, made eradication impossible." "Furthermore, while India has been polio-free for a year, there has been a huge increase in non-polio acute flaccid paralysis (NPAFP). In 2011, there were an extra 47,500 new cases of NPAFP. Clinically indistinguishable from polio paralysis but twice as deadly, the incidence of NPAFP was directly proportional to doses of oral polio received."

Correlation of Polio vaccine and Acute Flaccid Paralysis

Study title: Correlation between Non-Polio Acute Flaccid Paralysis Rates with Pulse Polio Frequency in India[141]; *International Journal if Environmental Research and Public Health, August 2018*

From the study: “From the results, the NPAFP rate has been shown to decline with a reduction in the pulse polio doses. This response to de-challenging adds weight to the likelihood of there being a causative association with OPV vaccinations.”

The following graph shows Non-polio AFP over the years in the state of UP alongside the 5-year cumulative doses of OPV.

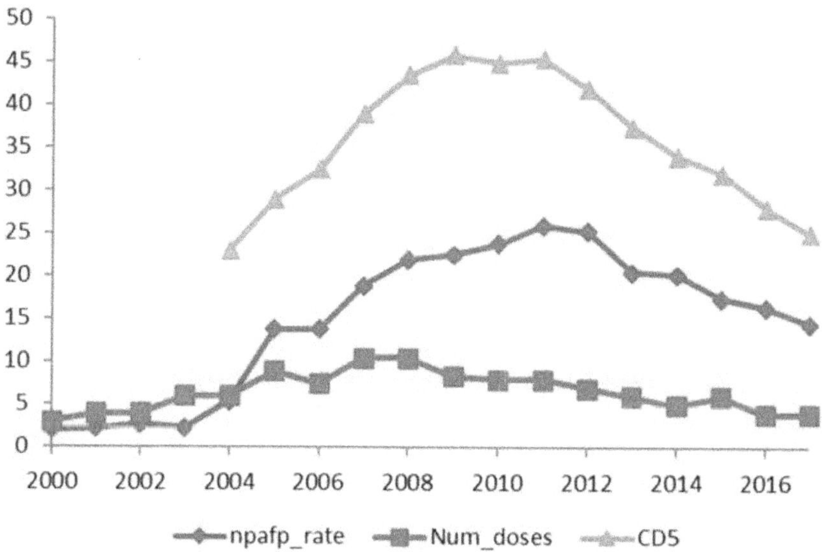

What can we understand from the above graph? You can see that as the doses of polio vaccine increased, more cases of acute flaccid paralysis were detected, and when the doses of polio vaccine decreased, less cases of AFP were detected, it shows a correlative of polio vaccine and paralysis.

THE VACCINE INJURY COMPENSATION PROGRAM

The National Vaccine Injury Compensation Program (NVICP) started in 1986, is a "court" that was created to compensate people injured by certain vaccines. To date they have paid out over 4 billion dollars in claims and attorney's fees for victims of vaccine injury. Since much of the cost of vaccines and vaccine programs are underwritten by our government, in a roundabout way we are all footing the bill.

"Since 1988, over 24,441 petitions have been filed with the Vaccine Injury Compensation Program (VICP). Over that 30-year time period, 20,300 petitions have been adjudicated, with 8,353 of those determined to be compensable, while 11,947 were dismissed. Total compensation paid over the life of the program is approximately $4.6 billion."[122]

Fiscal Year	Number of Compensated Awards	Petitioners' Award Amount	Attorneys' Fees/Costs Payments	Number of Payments to Attorneys (Dismissed Cases)	Attorneys' Fees/Costs Payments (Dismissed Cases)	Number of Payments to Interim Attorneys'	Interim Attorneys' Fees/Costs Payments	Total Outlays
FY 2016	689	$230,140,251.20	$16,298,140.59	99	$2,741,830.10	59	$3,502,709.91	$252,682,931.80
FY 2017	706	$252,245,932.78	$22,045,785.00	131	$4,439,538.57	52	$3,363,464.24	$282,094,720.59
FY 2018	521	$199,588,007.04	$16,658,440.14	112	$5,106,382.65	58	$5,151,148.78	$226,503,978.61
FY 2019	653	$196,217,707.64	$18,991,247.55	102	$4,791,157.52	65	$5,457,545.23	$225,457,657.94
FY 2020	733	$186,860,677.55	$20,165,357.38	113	$5,750,317.99	76	$5,090,482.24	$217,866,835.16
FY 2021	722	$210,447,660.77	$24,884,274.59	140	$6,942,253.81	54	$4,675,724.68	$246,949,913.85
Total	8,296	$4,281,609,631.73	$251,185,085.41	5,706	$97,587,743.30	619	$48,038,345.87	$4,678,420,806.31

The Government Bailed Out the Vaccine Industry

The National Childhood Vaccine Injury Act of 1986 protects vaccine manufacturers from lawsuits, i.e., the pharmaceutical companies cannot be sued for vaccine injuries or deaths. In the mid-1980s, the vaccine industry was facing the threat of bankruptcy, because of the large number of lawsuits brought by and won by vaccine injured individuals. So, rather than requiring the industry clean up their act, the government decided to require the complaints come before a special magistrate and the government defended against those complaints with government attorneys. Severe limits to awards were imposed and the complainants are required to prove their case, without the ability to subpoena records like they would in any other legal proceeding. Despite the cards being stacked against families of vaccine injured children, the "Vaccine Court" has awarded over 4 billion dollars to date!

Vaccines are the only class of drugs that have been given this special kind of protection. Think about it. Vaccines also are streamlined into production without the same scrutiny necessary for all other kinds of drugs and yet, vaccine manufacturers have no accountability for quality control. That is a recipe for disaster when they have no ramifications for inadequate safety studies, lack of long-term follow-up studies, sloppy manufacturing processes or poor-quality control.

Since the vaccine court has awarded $4.6 billion compensation for vaccine injured children, that certainly doesn't support the claim that vaccines are completely safe. You can see the amounts of petitions filed, the awards given, and the number of cases filed and compensated for each vaccine from Health Resources and Services Administration data. The flu vaccine is the most compensated vaccine amongst all.[122]

Petitions Filed, Compensated and Dismissed, by Alleged Vaccine, Since the Beginning of VICP, 10/01/1988 through 10/01/2021

Vaccines	Filed Injury	Filed Death	Filed Grand Total	Compensated	Dismissed
DTaP-IPV	16	0	16	5	4
DT	69	9	78	26	52
DTP	3,288	696	3,984	1,273	2,709
DTP-HIB	20	8	28	7	21
DTaP	479	86	565	245	268
DTaP-Hep B-IPV	97	39	136	44	64
DTaP-HIB	11	1	12	7	4
DTaP-IPV-HIB	50	21	71	17	39
Td	231	3	234	132	79
Tdap	1,052	8	1,060	542	117
Tetanus	170	3	173	87	48
Hepatitis A (Hep A)	134	7	141	62	39
Hepatitis B (Hep B)	737	62	799	288	442
Hep A-Hep B	42	0	42	22	9
Hep B-HIB	8	0	8	5	3
HIB	48	3	51	21	20
HPV	548	17	565	146	253
Influenza	7,916	200	8,116	4,367	787

PERSONAL, RELIGIOUS AND MEDICAL EXEMPTIONS

Personal Exemptions: This exemption is based on a person's right to decide what they will consent to. This is paramount to our freedoms. If we allow the government to force any medical procedure on us or our children, where will it stop? As you have seen in this document, there are forces that have put profits ahead of safety, power ahead of freedom. The argument that vaccines are for the greater good of society is worthless, because as The Vaccine Crime Report has proven, the science is far from settled. In fact, it's not even close! To take away our personal right to the sanctity of ours and our children's bodies, based on what we have seen in this Book is not only wrong, but also criminal.

Religious Exemptions: People of faith have a sincere and moral argument against vaccines and particularly the ones that contain DNA from aborted fetuses. The decision about one's conscious is between them and God. If it is based on the sanctity of life, and that life begins at conception, and that all life is precious because we are image bearers of God; there is no other position one can take. Many religions have valid reasons for refusing vaccine based on the teachings and value systems of their faith. They all have a right to exercise their faith based on our freedom of religion. "We the people" need to fight to keep that right!

Medical Exemptions: This is the last protection to stand after personal and religious exemptions are stripped away. This is where the battle lines are currently being drawn in several states. In many states, parents have lost personal belief exemptions. In many states, parents have lost religious exemptions. In the current climate of stripping rights of parents, to make health care decisions for their own children, the last right many have is the right to a medical exemption. Even that is under attack.

Doctors that write medical exemptions are under attack. Their livelihood is being threatened. Their practices are being destroyed. Well-meaning doctors, acting in the best interest of their patients are suffering for doing the right thing. The government has decided what is right for every child. They claim that neither the parents nor the doctors know the best of their children and thus force toxic medical procedures like vaccines on infants. When will the insanity end?

VACCINATIONS ARE EXTREMELY PROFITABLE

How much do the top vaccine manufacturers make per year?[145]

Merck & Co:
$6.750 billion in 2016
$7.545 billion (projected for 2023)

Glaxo Smith Kline:
$6.219 billion in 2016
$8.657 billion (projected for 2023)

Pfizer:
$6.071 billion in 2016
$7.133 billion (projected for 2023)

Sanofi:
$5.568 billion in 2016
$6.825 billion (projected for 2023)

Total:
$24.608 billion in 2016
$30.16 billion (projected for 2023)

CONCLUSION: WHAT IS THE NEXT STEP

As we have explored throughout this book, the science on vaccines is far from settled. Yet, it is unfortunate—and even tragic—that many people dismiss, ridicule, or outright refuse to question what they do not fully understand. Whether due to misinformation, blind faith in authority, or simple unwillingness to challenge their existing beliefs, this mindset has real consequences—not just for themselves but for their children and future generations. Why do so many resist looking deeper into this issue? Perhaps it's the discomfort of realizing that their long-held beliefs might be wrong. For doctors, acknowledging this truth would mean confronting the reality that they may have unknowingly misled their patients for years. That's not an easy thing to face. Pride, ego, and fear of professional or personal repercussions often prevent even well-intentioned individuals from questioning the status quo.

Governments, pharmaceutical companies, and many within the medical establishment continue to turn a blind eye—not because of a lack of evidence, but because there is simply too much at stake. The vaccine industry is a multi-billion-dollar enterprise with powerful financial incentives to sustain its narrative. For some, it's about preserving their reputation; for others, it's about protecting their careers. But for those at the top, it often comes down to one thing: money.

In a world where profit and power often take precedence over truth and public well-being, it is more important than ever to maintain a healthy level of skepticism. I urge you to question, investigate, and examine all sides of the argument. Do not accept claims—whether from the media, medical professionals, or government agencies—without seeking evidence for yourself. We have been given the intellect and reasoning ability to seek the truth. The answers are out there for those willing to look. My hope is that this book serves as a catalyst for deeper inquiry and critical thinking—because only by asking the hard questions can we ever hope to find real answers.

The children of the world deserve a champion that will fight for their right to live a full and unencumbered life, full of health, intellectual well-being, and the ability to contribute for themselves and society as a whole. The extent of the tragedy for millions of families dealing with everything from ADHD, learning disabilities, behavioral challenges, neurological deficits, autism spectrum disorders, allergies, eczema, asthma, autoimmune conditions, type 1 diabetes, rheumatoid arthritis, obesity, cancer, reproductive and thyroid issues and even death is unimaginable.

I urge every honest, pure-hearted individual—regardless of career, financial, or political consequences—to follow the evidence wherever it leads. Truth must take precedence over biased narratives. If you are not fully convinced that vaccines are entirely safe, effective, and delivering on their promises, then you must advocate for full transparency and an unbiased investigation into vaccine safety concerns. It is time to develop a different strategy to keep our children safe from disease and from overzealous special interests that profit from pumping toxins, chemicals, and foreign DNA into young bodies.

To those who choose to take a stand—thank you. Your willingness to question, investigate, and share this crucial message is the key to change. If this book has inspired you, let that inspiration drive action. Share this information widely. Speak up. Nothing changes unless enough people care enough to make it happen. You have the power to be part of that transformation. Now that you know the truth, your courage and conviction can help shape a healthier, safer world for millions today and for generations to come.

Request to doctors:

During their 8 to 12 years of medical education, doctors and pediatricians receive only minimal training on vaccines—often limited to just a few hours. This training does not focus on vaccine ingredients, potential side effects, or long-term safety studies. Instead, it primarily emphasizes how to encourage parents to comply with the "recommended" childhood vaccination schedule. As a result, many doctors have been conditioned to accept vaccine policies without question, prioritizing industry guidelines over independent scientific scrutiny. True medical inquiry demands an open, evidence-based approach—one that too many in the profession have been discouraged from pursuing.

Rather than blindly accepting what is spoon-fed to them, medical doctors must take responsibility for their own due diligence—seeking out the truth, no matter where it leads. If new and compelling evidence challenges long-held beliefs, the right course of action is to reassess and adapt. True integrity lies in the willingness to embrace truth over comfort, and only by doing so can one find peace, knowing they are standing on the side of what is right.

It's time for doctors to take the lead by dedicating time and effort to independently examine the evidence for themselves. Rather than relying solely on industry-driven guidelines, they should empower their patients with informed choices—reevaluating the vaccine schedule and eliminating unnecessary vaccinations where appropriate. Additionally, doctors must expand their knowledge of safe and natural alternatives, guiding patients toward a lifestyle that strengthens the immune system through proper nutrition, hydration, exercise, and stress management. True healthcare should prioritize prevention, informed decision-making, and overall well-being.

Request to humanity:

We urge every reader to share *The Vaccine Crime Report* within their community. The foundation of the medical-industrial complex relies on public ignorance—an uninformed society follows blindly, while an informed one questions, resists, and demands accountability. The most powerful action we can take is to spread awareness.

It is especially crucial to educate those in positions of influence—individuals who can help shape policies and public perception. Distribute *The Vaccine Crime Report* to school administrators and teachers, hospital directors and medical staff, law enforcement officers, lawyers and judges, pastors, mayors, commissioners, local media editors, and journalists. Knowledge is the catalyst for change, and when enough people understand the truth, the system can no longer operate unchecked.

This information must reach everyone in positions of public service. These individuals, often unknowingly, become enforcers of a system that harms millions—blindly following orders that result in widespread suffering, lifelong health damage, and even loss of life. However, ignorance is not an excuse. Once public servants truly understand the reality of what is happening, they will no longer serve as instruments of a corrupt system—unless they choose to be complicit. The time to act is now. Awareness leads to accountability, and only through informed action can we begin to dismantle this cycle of harm.

Now is the time to stand up for humanity. This is not just about raising awareness—it's about building a future where truth prevails over deception. We must come together to create new systems rooted in transparency, integrity, and genuine well-being. Be a beacon of light in a world overshadowed by misinformation. If good enough people take a stand, the future will be brighter than we can even begin to imagine.

THE SHOCKING TRUTH OF PARACETAMOL

The Shocking Truth of Paracetamol gives you access to the findings of credible scientific studies published in prestigious medical journals that refute the claim that paracetamol is safe and effective. The health complications associated with paracetamol are asthma, liver failure, kidney failure, debilitating chronic diseases, impaired neurodevelopment, etc. This book also serves as a guide to manage fever and flu without drugs to avoid future health issues.

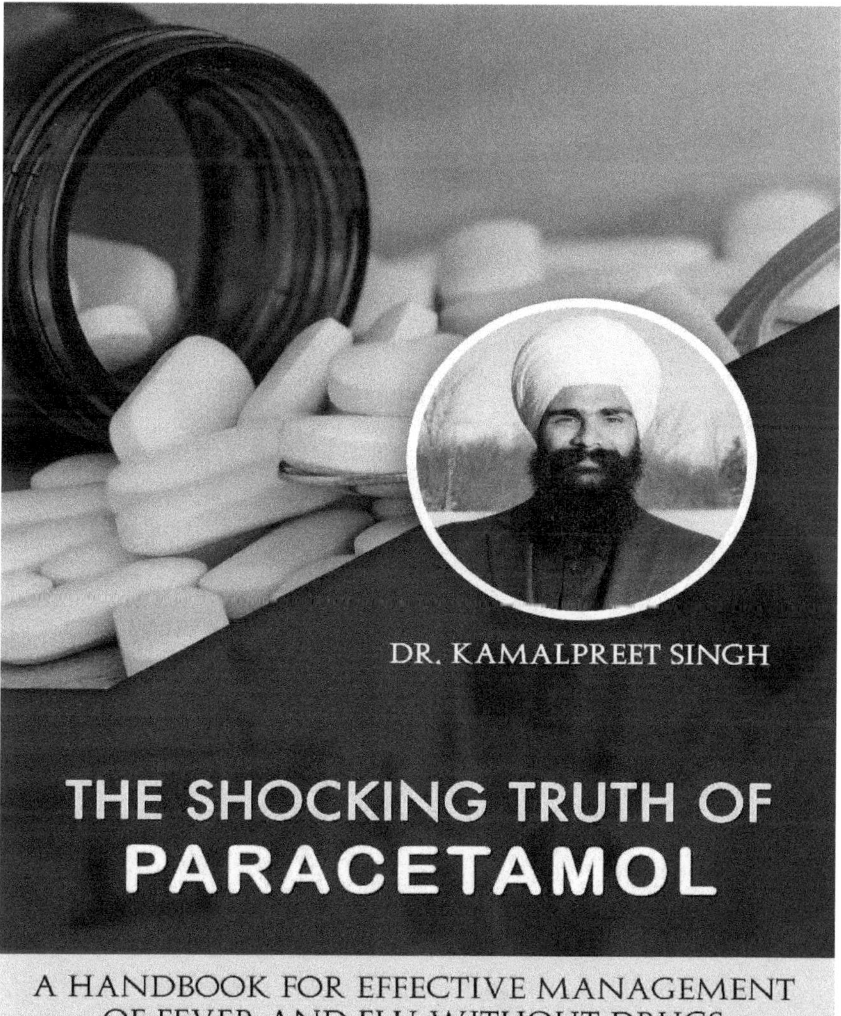

DO FACE MASKS REALLY WORK?

There is no scientific evidence that can conclude the benefits of wearing a face mask. At the same time, a plethora of evidence suggests that wearing face masks for longer duration can cause hypoxia, hypercapnia, headaches, breathing difficulties, cardiovascular implications and nervous system changes leading to exacerbation of existing chronic diseases, especially asthma, bronchitis, migraines, and Obstructive Pulmonary Disorder.

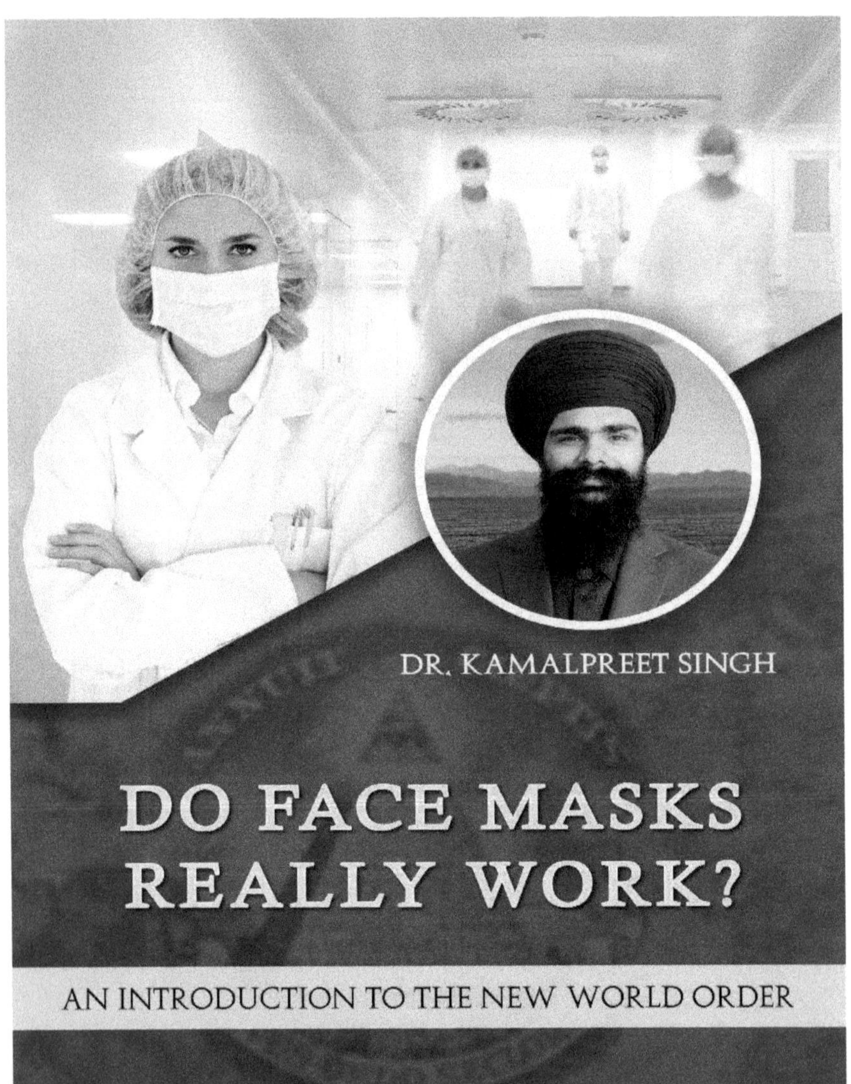

POSH WAY TO REVERSE TYPE 2 DIABETES

Diabetes is believed to be irreversible by the medical industry. The patient is expected to be on medications forever with an ever-increasing list of health complications including vision loss, heart disease, and kidney failure. "P.O.S.H. Way to Reverse Type-2 and Type-1 Diabetes" expounds self-healing methods to regulate blood sugar naturally. It leads to diabetes reversal and elimination of medications gradually. The book can be purchased from Amazon or through the website https://gosatvik.ca

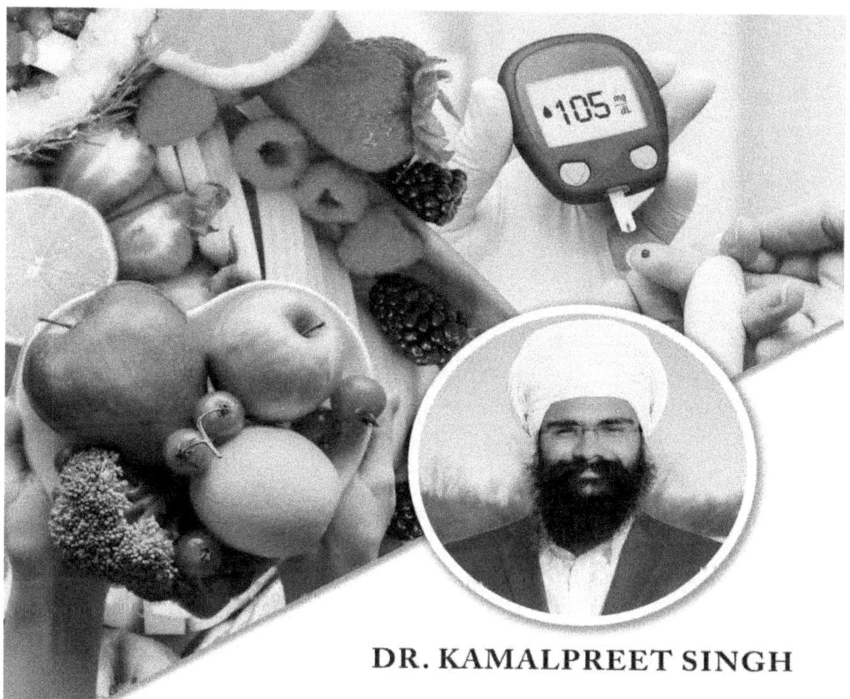

P.O.S.H. WAY TO REVERSE
TYPE 2 & TYPE 1
DIABETES

PROTOCOL OF SELF HEALING FOR
REVERSING DIABETES WITHOUT DRUGS

ADVANCED NUTRITION THERAPY

Advanced Nutrition Therapy: Goodbye Drugs and Diseases is a Best-Selling book by Dr. Kamalpreet Singh that focuses on reversal of chronic illness through whole food plant-based diet. Delicious and easy to make recipes are provided to ensure healthy cooking habits. The book was rated in top 5 book in Diabetes section by Amazon. Thousands of copies of the book have been sold within few months of publishing. The book can be purchased from Amazon or through the website https://gosatvik.ca

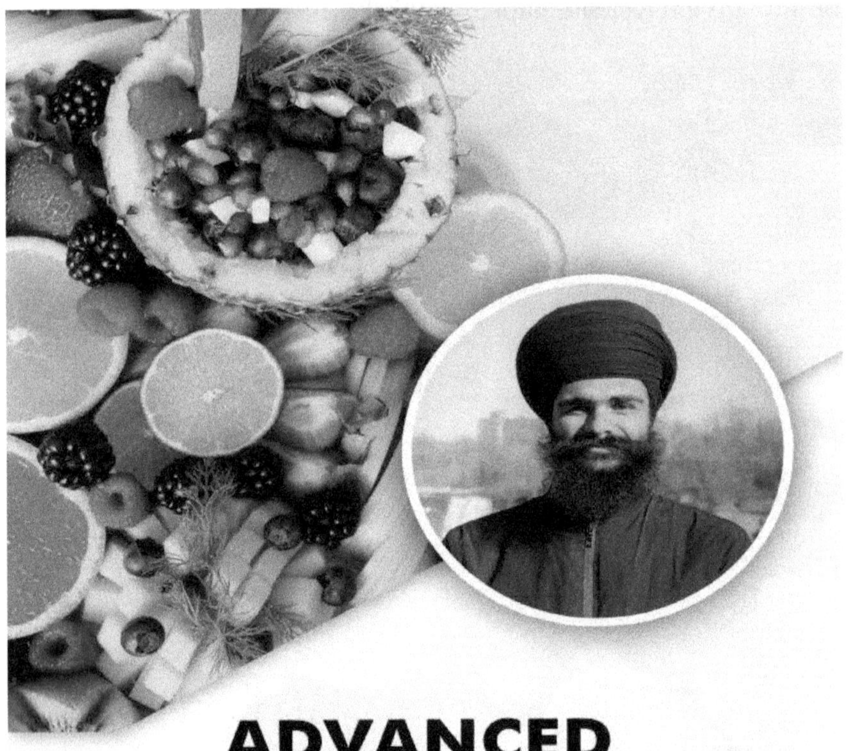

ADVANCED NUTRITION THERAPY

Goodbye Drugs and Diseases

Dr. Kamalpreet Singh

NO MORE DIABETES | NO MORE HYPERTENSION

REFERENCES

1. Linda T. Kohn "*To Err Is Human; To Fail to Improve Is Unconscionable*" Institute of Medicine (1999), https://www.supersalud.gob.cl/observatorio/671/articles-14460_recurso_1.pdf

2. Barbara Starfield MD "*Is US Health Really the Best in the World*" Journal of the American Medical Association (2000), https://www.jhsph.edu/research/centers-and-institutes/johns-hopkins-primary-care-policy-center/Publications_PDFs/A154.pdf

3. Gary Null PhD "*Death by Medicine*" (2011), https://advancedmedicine.ca/wp-content/uploads/2013/09/How-Effective-is-Modern-Medicine.pdf

4. John T. James PhD "*A New Evidence-based Estimate of Patient Harms Associated with Hospital Care*", Journal of Public Safety (2013), https://journals.lww.com/journalpatientsafety/Fulltext/2013/09000/A_New,_Evidence_based_Estimate_of_Patient_Harms.2.aspx

5. Brianna A. da Silva MD "*The alarming reality of medication error a patient case and review of Pennsylvania and National data*" Journal of Community Hospital Internal Medicine Perspectives (2016), https://www.ncbi.nlm.nih.gov/pmc/articles/PMC5016741/

6. Kevin Trudeau "*Natural Cures They Don't Want You To Know About*" (2006), https://www.amazon.ca/Natural-Cures-They-Dont-About/dp/0975599593

7. Martha N. Gardner PhD "*The Doctors' Choice Is America's Choice*" American Journal of Public health (2006), https://www.ncbi.nlm.nih.gov/pmc/articles/PMC1470496/

8. Wikipedia "*Thalidomide*", https://en.wikipedia.org/wiki/Thalidomide

9. Dr Vernon Coleman MB ChB DSc FRSA "*Anyone Who Tells You Vaccines Are Safe and Effective is Lying*" (2019), https://www.amazon.ca/Anyone-Tells-Vaccines-Effective-Lying/dp/1091757712

10. "*2016 Performance Recognition Program*" Blue Cross Blue Shield Blue Care Network of Michigan (2016), http://www.whale.to/c/2016-BCN-BCBSM-Incentive-Program-Booklet.pdf

11. Dr. Raymond Obomsawin, Ph.D. "*Disease decline before introduction of immunisation*", http://www.whale.to/vaccines/decline1.html

12. Dr. Suzanne Humphries "*Vaccination*", http://drsuzanne.net/dr-suzanne-humphries-vaccines-vaccination/

13. Thomas S. Cowan MD "*The Contagion Myth: Why Viruses (including "Coronavirus") Are Not the Cause of Disease*" (2020), https://www.goodreads.com/en/book/show/54786062-the-contagion-myth

14. Dr. Kamalpreet Singh "*Advanced Nutrition Therapy: Goodbye Drugs and Diseases*" (2022), https://gosatvik.ca/books/

15. Huaidong Du "*Fresh fruit consumption in relation to incident diabetes and diabetic vascular complications: A 7-y prospective study of 0.5 million Chinese adults*" PLoS Medicine (2017), https://www.ncbi.nlm.nih.gov/pmc/articles/PMC5388466/

16. Paul S. Fishman "*Immunization does not interfere with uptake and transport by motor neurons of the binding fragment of tetanus toxin*" Journal of Neuroscience Research (2006), https://pubmed.ncbi.nlm.nih.gov/16557581/

17. Ann Brenoff "*The Elderly Are Taking Too Many Pills*" HuffPost (2017), https://www.huffingtonpost.com/ann-brenoff/elderly-taking-too-many-pills_b_7079060.html

18. Melissa Conrad Stoppler MD "*The Most Common Medication Errors*" MedicineNet, https://www.medicinenet.com/drugs_the_most_common_medication_errors/views.htm

19. Naru Zhang "*Recent advances in the development of vaccines for chronic inflammatory autoimmune diseases*" Vaccine (2018), https://pubmed.ncbi.nlm.nih.gov/29706295/

20. "*Vaccine Excipient Summary: Excipients Included in U.S. Vaccines*" CDC (2021), https://www.cdc.gov/vaccines/pubs/pinkbook/downloads/appendices/b/excipient-table-2.pdf

21. "*Peer-Reviewed, Published Research Showing Adverse Effects of Mercury*" Children's Health Defense, https://childrenshealthdefense.org/wp-content/uploads/mercury-all-sources-research-combined-chd.pdf

22. D.A. Geier "*Mitochondrial dysfunction, impaired oxidative-reduction activity, degeneration, and death in human neuronal and fetal cells induced by low-level exposure to thimerosal and other metal compounds*" Journal of Toxicological and Environmental Chemistry (2009), https://www.ncbi.nlm.nih.gov/pmc/articles/PMC3924342/

23. David A. Geier "*Thimerosal: clinical, epidemiologic, and biochemical studies*" International Journal of Clinical Chemistry (2015), https://pubmed.ncbi.nlm.nih.gov/25708367/

24. L. A. Sealey "*Environmental factors in the development of autism spectrum disorders*" Journal of Environment International (2016), https://www.ncbi.nlm.nih.gov/pubmed/26826339

25. Esther A. Coors "*Nipple cream warning: harmful to nursing infants*" ScienceBlogs (2008), https://scienceblogs.com/terrasig/2008/05/25/nipple-cream-warning-harmful-t

26. "*Polysorbate 80 in medical products and nonimmunologic anaphylactoid reactions*" Annals of Allergy, Asthma & Immunology (2005), https://www.ncbi.nlm.nih.gov/pubmed/16400901

27. "*List of classifications by cancer sites with sufficient or limited evidence in humans, IARC Monographs Volumes 1–132a*" International Agency for Research on Cancer (2019), https://monographs.iarc.who.int/wp-content/uploads/2019/07/Classifications_by_cancer_site.pdf

28. Wikipedia "*beta-Propiolactone*", https://en.wikipedia.org/wiki/Beta-Propiolactone#cite_note-nih-2

29. US Department of Health and Human Services "*beta-Propiolactone*" Report on Carcinogens, National Toxicology Program, Thirteenth Edition (2014), https://ntp.niehs.nih.gov/ntp/roc/content/profiles/propiolactone.pdf

30. "*Occupational Safety and Health Guideline for Beta-Propiolactone*" CDC, https://www.cdc.gov/niosh/docs/81-123/pdfs/0528.pdf

31. New Jersey Department of Health and Senior Services, "*Hazardous Substances Fact Sheet: Beta-Propiolactone*" (2002), https://www.nj.gov/health/eoh/rtkweb/documents/fs/0228.pdf

32. Scott M. Ravis "*Glutaraldehyde-induced and formaldehyde-induced allergic contact dermatitis among dental hygienists and assistants*" Journal of American Dental Association (2003), https://pubmed.ncbi.nlm.nih.gov/12956347/

33. Material Safety Data Sheet (MSDS) "*Phenol*" Sigma-Aldrich (2020), https://www.sigmaaldrich.com/CA/en/sds/sial/p5566

34. "*International and national regulations and guidelines pertinent to human exposure to phenol*" CDC, https://www.atsdr.cdc.gov/toxprofiles/tp115-c8.pdf

35. Xu Jie "*Neurotoxic effects of nonylphenol: a review*" Wiener klinische Wochenschrift (2013), https://www.ncbi.nlm.nih.gov/pubmed/23334477

36. Material Safety Data Sheet "*Cetyltrimethylammonium Bromide*", https://datasheets.scbt.com/sc-278833.pdf

37. "*Gentamicin sulfate injection Warnings and Precautions*" Pfizer, https://www.pfizermedicalinformation.com/en-us/gentamicin/warnings

38. Barbro C. Carlson "*The Endogenous Adjuvant Squalene Can Induce a Chronic T-Cell-Mediated Arthritis in Rats*" American Journal of Pathology (2000), https://www.ncbi.nlm.nih.gov/pmc/articles/PMC1850095/

39. Joanne Waldron "*Rat Poison Chemical Found GARDASIL*" (2008), http://www.offtheradar.co.nz/vaccines/104-rat-poison-chemical-in-gardasil.html/

40. Anne Riederer ScD "*BORAX - Summary of Health Risks Associated with Using Borax in Artisanal and Small-Scale Gold Mining*" Blacksmith Institute (2013), http://www.pureearth.org/wp-content/uploads/2021/03/Borax-in-ASGM-Final-April-1-2013.pdf

41. "*ACAM2000, (Smallpox (Vaccinia) Vaccine, Live)*" FDA, https://www.fda.gov/media/75792/download

42. Kyle Keinath "*Myocarditis secondary to smallpox vaccination*" British Medical Journal Case Reports (2018), https://www.ncbi.nlm.nih.gov/pmc/articles/PMC5878341/

43. Antonietta M Gatti "*New Quality-Control Investigations on Vaccines: Micro- and Nano contamination*" Internation Journal of Vaccines and Vaccination (2017), http://medcraveonline.com/IJVV/IJVV-04-00072.php

44. "*PER.C6 Cell Lines*" Creative Biolabs, http://www.gmp-creativebiolabs.com/per-c6-cell-lines_74.htm

45. Bo Ma "*Characteristics and viral propagation properties of a new human diploid cell line, walvax-2, and its suitability as a candidate cell substrate for vaccine production*" Human Vaccines and Immunotherapeutics (2015), https://www.ncbi.nlm.nih.gov/pmc/articles/PMC4526020/#cit0007

46. "*The Ethics of The Walvax-2 Cell Strain*" Nebraska Coalition for Ethical Research, http://ethicalresearch.net/positions/the-ethics-of-the-walvax-2-cell-strain/

47. Dr. Theresa A. Deisher "*Impact of environmental factors on the prevalence of autistic disorder after 1979*" Journal of Public Health and Epidemiology (2014), https://academicjournals.org/journal/JPHE/article-full-text-pdf/C98151247042

48. Dr. Theresa A. Deisher "*Epidemiologic and Molecular Relationship Between Vaccine Manufacture and Autism Spectrum Disorder Prevalence*" Issues in Law and Medicine (2015), https://pubmed.ncbi.nlm.nih.gov/26103708/

49. Jessica Farnsworth, M.D. "*DEVELOPMENT OF VACCINES FROM ABORTED BABIES*" Eternal Perspective Ministries (2011), https://www.epm.org/static/uploads/downloads/Vaccines_Using_Tissue_from_Aborted_Babies.pdf

50. "*Cumulative Analysis of Post-authorization Adverse Event Reports*" Pfizer (2021), https://phmpt.org/wp-content/uploads/2021/11/5.3.6-postmarketing-experience.pdf

51. Dr. Biswaroop R. Chowdhury "*NICE Way to Cure COVID-19*" (2020), https://biswaroop.com/nicebook

52. "*VAERS COVID Vaccine Mortality Reports*" Vaccine Adverse Event Reporting System, https://openvaers.com/covid-data/mortality

53. Lazarus Ross MBBS *"Electronic Support for Public Health–Vaccine Adverse Event Reporting System (ESP:VAERS)"* (2011), https://digital.ahrq.gov/sites/default/files/docs/publication/r18hs017045-lazarus-final-report-2011.pdf

54. Piero Olliaro "*COVID-19 vaccine efficacy and effectiveness – the elephant (not) in the room"* The Lancet (2021), https://www.thelancet.com/journals/lanmic/article/PIIS2666-5247(21)00069-0/fulltext

55. Naama Lessans MD "*The effect of BNT162b2 SARS-CoV-2 mRNA vaccine on menstrual cycle symptoms in healthy women*"; International Journal of Gynecology & Obstetrics (2022), https://obgyn.onlinelibrary.wiley.com/doi/pdf/10.1002/ijgo.14356

56. Rachael Bailey "*Incidence of Autoimmune Arthritis Disease Flare Following SARS-CoV-2 Vaccination and its Association with Concurrent NSAID Use*" IJDRP (2022), https://ijdrp.org/index.php/ijdrp/article/view/323

57. Sintaroo Watanabe "*SARS-CoV-2 vaccine and increased myocarditis mortality risk: A population based comparative study in Japan*" MedArchive (2022), https://www.medrxiv.org/content/10.1101/2022.10.13.22281036v1

58. Paul Thomas MD "*Relative Incidence of Office Visits and Cumulative Rates of Billed Diagnoses Along the Axis of Vaccination*"; International Journal of Environmental Research and Public Health (2020), https://www.ar25.org/sites/default/files/ijerph-17-08674-v3.pdf

59. Anthony Mawson "*Pilot comparative study on the health of vaccinated and unvaccinated 6-to 12-year-old U.S. children*"; Journal of Translational Science (2017), https://www.researchgate.net/publication/317086531_Pilot_comparative_study_on_the_health_of_vaccinated_and_unvaccinated_6-to_12-year-old_US_children

60. Neil Z. Miller "*Combining Childhood Vaccines at One Visit Is Not Safe*"; American Physicians and Surgeons (2016), https://www.jpands.org/vol21no2/miller.pdf

61. Jason M Glanz "*A population-based cohort study of undervaccination in 8 managed care organizations across the United States*"; *Journal of American Medical Association Pediatrics (2013),* https://pubmed.ncbi.nlm.nih.gov/23338829/

62. Neil Z. Miller "*Infant mortality rates regressed against number of vaccine doses routinely given: Is there a biochemical or synergistic toxicity?*" Human and Experimental Toxicology (2011), https://www.ncbi.nlm.nih.gov/pmc/articles/PMC3170075/

63. Kristina Kristen "*Japan Leads the Way: No Vaccine Mandates and No MMR Vaccine = Healthier Children in Japan*" Children's Health Defense (2019), https://childrenshealthdefense.org/news/vaccines/japan-leads-the-way-no-vaccine-mandates-and-no-mmr-vaccine-healthier-children/

64. Pedro L. Moro MD "Adverse events following Haemophilus influenzae type b vaccines in the Vaccine Adverse Event Reporting System, 1990-2013"; The Journal of Pediatrics (2015), https://www.ncbi.nlm.nih.gov/pmc/articles/PMC6500451/

65. B. Zinka "*Unexplained cases of sudden infant death shortly after hexavalent vaccination*" Vaccine (2006), https://www.researchgate.net/publication/7833641_Unexplained_cases_of_sudden_infant_death_shortly_after_hexavalent_vaccination

66. Rüdiger von Kries "*Sudden and unexpected deaths after the administration of hexavalent vaccines (diphtheria, tetanus, pertussis, poliomyelitis, hepatitis B, Haemophilius influenzae type b): is there a signal?*" European Journal of Pediatrics (2005), https://pubmed.ncbi.nlm.nih.gov/15602672/

67. D. A. Treffert "*Epidemiology of Infantile Autism*" Archives of General Psychiatry (1970), https://pubmed.ncbi.nlm.nih.gov/5436867/

68. L Burd "*A Prevalence Study of Pervasive Developmental Disorders in North Dakota*" Journal of the American Academy of Child and Adolescent Psychiatry (1987), https://pubmed.ncbi.nlm.nih.gov/3499432/

69. "*Data & Statistics on Autism Spectrum Disorder*" CDC, https://www.cdc.gov/ncbddd/autism/data.html

70. "*Autism and Vaccines Around the World: Vaccine Schedules, Autism Rates, and Under 5 Mortality*" Generation Rescue Inc. (2009), http://www.rescuepost.com/files/gr-autism_and_vaccines_world_special_report1.pdf

71. Stephanie Seneff "*Empirical Data Confirm Autism Symptoms Related to Aluminum and Acetaminophen Exposure*", Entropy (2012), https://www.mdpi.com/1099-4300/14/11/2227/pdf

72. William Shaw, Ph.D. "*Evidence that Increased Acetaminophen use in Genetically Vulnerable Children Appears to be a Major Cause of the Epidemics of Autism, Attention Deficit with Hyperactivity, and Asthma*"; The Great Plains Laboratory (2015), https://www.greatplainslaboratory.com/articles-1/2015/11/13/evidence-that-increased-acetaminophen-use-in-genetically-vulnerable-children-appears-to-be-a-major-cause-of-the-epidemics-of-autism-attention-deficit-with-hyperactivity-and-asthma

73. Dr. Theresa A. Deisher "*Impact of Environmental Factors on the Prevalence of Autistic Disorder after 1979*"; Public Health and Epidemiology (2014), http://www.academicjournals.org/journal/JPHE/article-full-text/C98151247042

74. Lucija Tomljenovic "*Autism Spectrum Disorders and Aluminum Vaccine Adjuvants*"; A Comprehensive Guide to Autism (2014), https://link.springer.com/referenceworkentry/10.1007%2F978-1-4614-4788-7_89

75. José G Dórea "*Low-dose Thimerosal in pediatric vaccines: Adverse effects in perspective*"; Environmental Research (2017), https://www.ncbi.nlm.nih.gov/pubmed/?term=27816865

76. D. A. Geier "*A comprehensive review of mercury provoked autism*"; Indian Journal of Medical Research (2008), https://www.ncbi.nlm.nih.gov/pubmed/?term=19106436

77. Heather A. Young "*Thimerosal exposure in infants and neurodevelopmental disorders: an assessment of computerized medical records in the Vaccine Safety Datalink*"; Journal of the Neurological Sciences (2008), https://www.ncbi.nlm.nih.gov/pubmed/18482737

78. D. A. Geier "*A comparative evaluation of the effects of MMR immunization and mercury doses from thimerosal-containing childhood vaccines on the population prevalence of autism*" Medical Science Monitor (2004) https://www.ncbi.nlm.nih.gov/pubmed/?term=14976450

79. C. A. Shaw "*Aluminum in the central nervous system (CNS): toxicity in humans and animals, vaccine adjuvants, and autoimmunity*"; Immunologic Research (2013), https://www.ncbi.nlm.nih.gov/pubmed/?term=23609067

80. Guido Crisponi "*The meaning of aluminium exposure on human health and aluminium-related diseases*" Biomolecular Concepts (2013), https://www.ncbi.nlm.nih.gov/pubmed/?term=25436567

81. Stephen C. Bondy "*Prolonged exposure to low levels of aluminum leads to changes associated with brain aging and neurodegeneration*" Toxicology (2014), https://www.ncbi.nlm.nih.gov/pubmed/24189189

82. Gerwyn Morris "*The putative role of environmental aluminium in the development of chronic neuropathology in adults and children.*" Metabolic Brain Disease (2017), https://www.ncbi.nlm.nih.gov/pmc/articles/PMC5596046/

83. Nicholas J. Bishop MD "*Aluminum Neurotoxicity and Preterm Infants Receiving Intravenous Feeding Solutions*" New England Journal of Medicine (1997), http://www.nejm.org/doi/full/10.1056/NEJM199705293362203#t=article

84. "*Package Inserts & FDA Product Approvals*" FDA, https://www.immunize.org/fda/#hepb, https://gskpro.com/content/dam/global/hcpportal/en_US/Prescribing_Information/Engerix-B/pdf/ENGERIX-B.PDF

85. "*CFR - Code of Federal Regulations Title 21*" FDA (2022), http://www.accessdata.fda.gov/scripts/cdrh/cfdocs/cfcfr/CFRSearch.cfm?fr=201.323

86. Mike Adams "*EXCLUSIVE: Natural News tests flu vaccine for heavy metals, finds 25,000 times higher mercury level than EPA limit for water*" (2014), http://www.naturalnews.com/045418_flu_shots_influenza_vaccines_mercury.html

87. Muhammad U. Ijaz "*A study on the potential reprotoxic effects of thimerosal in male albino rats*" SJBS (2020), https://www.ncbi.nlm.nih.gov/pmc/articles/PMC7499386/

88. David A. Geier "*Thimerosal exposure & increasing trends of premature puberty in the vaccine safety datalink*", IJMR (2010), https://pubmed.ncbi.nlm.nih.gov/20424300/

89. "*Influenza A (H1N1) 2009 Monovalent Vaccine*" Sanofi (2009), https://www.fda.gov/downloads/biologicsbloodvaccines/vaccines/approvedproducts/ucm182404.pdf

90. "*Use of Influenza A (H1N1) 2009 Monovalent Vaccine, Recommendations of the Advisory Committee on Immunization Practices (ACIP)*" CDC (2009), https://www.cdc.gov/mmwr/preview/mmwrhtml/rr5810a1.htm

91. "*FDA Admits That Government Is Recommending Untested, Unlicensed Vaccines for Pregnant Women*" Children's Health Defense (2019), https://childrenshealthdefense.org/news/fda-admits-that-government-is-recommending-untested-unlicensed-vaccines-for-pregnant-women/

92. James G. Donahue "*Association of spontaneous abortion with receipt of inactivated influenza vaccine containing H1N1pdm09 in 2010-11 and 2011-12*" Vaccine (2017), https://www.ncbi.nlm.nih.gov/pmc/articles/PMC6501798/

93. T. Kemp "*Is infant immunization a risk factor for childhood asthma or allergy?*" Epidemiology (1997), https://www.ncbi.nlm.nih.gov/pubmed/9345669

94. Neil Z. Miller "*Analysis of health outcomes in vaccinated and unvaccinated children: Developmental delays, asthma, ear infections and gastrointestinal disorders*" Sage Open Medicine (2020), https://journals.sagepub.com/doi/10.1177/2050312120925344

95. J. Wahlberg "*Vaccinations may induce diabetes-related autoantibodies in one-year-old children*" Annals of the New York Academy of Sciences (2003), https://www.ncbi.nlm.nih.gov/pubmed/?term=14679101

96. John B. Classen MD "*Prevalence of Autism is Positively Associated with the Incidence of Type 1 Diabetes, but Negatively Associated with the Incidence of Type 2 Diabetes, Implication for the Etiology of the Autism Epidemic*" Open Access Scientific Reports (2013), https://www.omicsonline.org/scientific-reports/2155-9899-SR-679.pdf

97. John B. Classen MD "*Risk of Vaccine Induced Diabetes in Children with a Family History of Type 1 Diabetes*" The Open Pediatric Medicine Journal (2008), https://openpediatricmedicinejournal.com/contents/volumes/V2/TOPEDJ-2-7/TOPEDJ-2-7.pdf

98. John B. Classen MD "*Vaccines and the risk of insulin-dependent diabetes (IDDM): potential mechanism of action*" Medical Hypotheses (2001), https://pubmed.ncbi.nlm.nih.gov/11735306/

99. John B. Classen MD "*Review of Vaccine Induced Immune Overload and the Resulting Epidemics of Type 1 Diabetes and Metabolic Syndrome, Emphasis on Explaining the Recent Accelerations in the Risk of Prediabetes and other Immune Mediated Diseases*" Journal of Molecular and Genetic Medicine (2014), https://www.omicsonline.org/open-access/vaccine-induced-immune-overload-and-the-resulting-epidemics-of-type-diabetes-and-metabolic-syndrome-1747-0862.S1-025.php?aid=24058

100. Julie Mouchet "*Central Demyelinating Diseases after Vaccination Against Hepatitis B Virus: A Disproportionality Analysis within the VAERS Database*" Drug Safety (2018), https://www.ncbi.nlm.nih.gov/pubmed/29560597

101. Frederica Perera "*Prenatal environmental exposures, epigenetics, and disease*" Reproductive Toxicology (2011), *https://www.ncbi.nlm.nih.gov/pmc/articles/PMC3171169/*

102. Gayle Delong "*A positive association found between autism prevalence and childhood vaccination uptake across the U.S. population*" Journal of Toxicology and Environmental Health (2011), https://www.ncbi.nlm.nih.gov/pubmed/21623535

103. David A. Geier "*Thimerosal-containing Hepatitis B Vaccine Exposure is Highly Associated with Childhood Obesity: A Case-control Study Using the Vaccine Safety Datalink*" North American Journal of Medical Sciences (2016), https://www.ncbi.nlm.nih.gov/pmc/articles/PMC4982359/

104. C. M. Benjamin "*Joint and limb symptoms in children after immunisation with measles, mumps, and rubella vaccine*"; British Medical Journal (1992), https://pubmed.ncbi.nlm.nih.gov/1586818/

105. Yong-Shik Park "*Clinical Features of Post-Vaccination Guillain-Barré Syndrome (GBS) in Korea*" Journal of Korean Medical Science (2017), https://www.ncbi.nlm.nih.gov/pmc/articles/PMC5461320/

106. Marco Tulio Zanettini "*Pericarditis. Series of 84 consecutive cases*" Arquivos Brasileiros de Cardiologia (2004), https://www.ncbi.nlm.nih.gov/pubmed/?term=15320556

107. Danuta M. Skowronski "*Association between the 2008—09 seasonal influenza vaccine and pandemic HINI illness during Spring— summer 2009: four observational studies from Canada*" PLoS Medicine (2010), http://journals.plos.org/plosmedicine/article?id=10.1371/journal.pmed.1000258

108. Sharon Rikin "*Assessment of temporally-related acute respiratory illness following influenza vaccination*" Vaccine (2018), https://www.ncbi.nlm.nih.gov/pubmed/?term=29525279

109. Benjamin J. Cowling "*Increased Risk of Non-influenza Respiratory Virus Infections Associated with Receipt of Inactivated Influenza Vaccine*" Clinical Infectious Diseases (2012), https://www.ncbi.nlm.nih.gov/pmc/articles/PMC3404712/

110. Peter G. Szilagyi "*Influenza vaccine effectiveness among children 6 to 59 months of age during 2 influenza seasons: a case-cohort study*" Archives of Pediatrics and Adolescent Medicine (2008), https://www.ncbi.nlm.nih.gov/pubmed/?term=18838647

111. Kristina Rebelo "*Flu Vaccination May Triple Risk for Flu-Related Hospitalization in Children with Asthma*" American Thoracic Society International Conference (2009), https://www.medscape.com/viewarticle/703235

112. Vittorio Demicheli "*Vaccines for preventing influenza in healthy adults*" The Cochrane Database of Systematic Reviews (2018), https://www.cochranelibrary.com/cdsr/doi/10.1002/14651858.CD001269.pub6/full

113. Sue Corrigan "*Former science chief: 'MMR fears coming true*'" Daily Mail (2016), http://www.dailymail.co.uk/health/article-376203/Former-science-chief-MMR-fears-coming-true.html

114. "*CDC Whistleblower and Corruption*" A Voice for Choice, http://avoiceforchoice.org/cdcwhistleblower/

115. Dr. Alan Palmer "*1200 Studies- Truth Will Prevail eBook*" Wellnessdoc – Health and Lifestyle Coaching, https://www.wellnessdoc.com/1200studies/

116. "*Reported Measles Cases and Death per 100,000 population*" US (1912-1975), https://childhealthsafety.files.wordpress.com/2009/01/measlesmortalityusa1971-75_1.jpg

117. "Measles – Mortality Per 55 million all ages – England and Wales" 20th Century Mortality – Office for National Statistics (1901-1999), https://childhealthsafety.files.wordpress.com/2009/01/0707275measleslog.jpg

118. "*Measles Disease & Vaccine Information*" National Vaccine Information Center (2019), https://www.nvic.org/vaccines-and-diseases/measles/measles-vaccine-injury-death.aspx

119. G. A. Poland "*Failure to reach the goal of measles elimination. Apparent paradox of measles infections in immunized persons*" Archives of Internal Medicine (1994), https://www.ncbi.nlm.nih.gov/pubmed/?term=8053748

120. Gaston De Serres "*Largest measles epidemic in North America in a decade--Quebec, Canada, 2011*" Journal of Infectious Diseases (2013), https://www.ncbi.nlm.nih.gov/pubmed/?term=23264672

121. "Events Reported to VAERS After HPV Vaccines" Sanevax (2020), https://sanevax.org/wp-content/uploads/2020/01/Dec-2019.pdf

122. "*National Vaccine Injury Compensation Program - Monthly Statistics Report*" Health Resource and Service Administration data and statistics (2021), https://www.hrsa.gov/sites/default/files/hrsa/vaccine-compensation/data/data-statistics-report.pdf

123. Lucija Tomljenovic "*Human papillomavirus (HPV) vaccine policy and evidence-based Medicine: are they at odds?*" Annals of Medicine (2013), https://pubmed.ncbi.nlm.nih.gov/22188159/

124. Xianfang C.Liu "*Adverse events following HPV vaccination, Alberta 2006–2014*" Vaccine (2016), http://www.sciencedirect.com/science/article/pii/S0264410X16002036

125. Gayle DeLong "*A lowered probability of pregnancy in females in the USA aged 25-29 who received a human papillomavirus vaccine injection*" Journal of Toxicology and Environmental Health (2018), https://www.ncbi.nlm.nih.gov/pubmed/?term=29889622

126. Lance D. Johanson "*Court ruling confirms Gardasil vaccine kills people… scientific evidence beyond any doubt… so where is the outcry?*" Natural News (2018) https://www.naturalnews.com/2018-04-05-court-ruling-confirms-gardasil-vaccine-kills-people-scientific-evidence-beyond-any-doubt.html

127. Søren Wengel Mogensen "*The Introduction of Diphtheria-Tetanus-Pertussis and Oral Polio Vaccine Among Young Infants in an Urban African Community: A Natural Experiment*" E BioMedicine (2017), https://www.ncbi.nlm.nih.gov/pmc/articles/PMC5360569/

128. E. L. Hurwitz "*Effects of diphtheria-tetanus-pertussis or tetanus vaccination on allergies and allergy-related respiratory symptoms among children and adolescents in the United States*" Journal of Manipulative and Physiological Therapeutics (2000), https://pubmed.ncbi.nlm.nih.gov/10714532/

129. C. L. Cody "*Nature and rates of adverse reactions associated with DTP and DT immunizations in infants and children*" Pediatrics (1981), https://www.ncbi.nlm.nih.gov/pubmed/7031583

130. "*Tetanus Surveillance --- United States, 2001—2008*" Morbidity and Mortality Weekly Report CDC (2011), https://www.cdc.gov/mmwr/preview/mmwrhtml/mm6012a1.htm

131. "*Flash Facts About Lightning*" National Geographic (2005), https://news.nationalgeographic.com/news/2004/06/flash-facts-about-lightning/

132. Joanne Faryon "*Immunized People Getting Whooping Cough*" KPBS San Diego (2014), http://www.kpbs.org/news/2014/jun/12/immunized-people-getting-whooping-cough/

133. Carolyn M Gallagher "*Hepatitis B vaccination of male neonates and autism diagnosis, NHIS 1997-2002*" Journal of Toxicology and Environmental Health (2010), https://pubmed.ncbi.nlm.nih.gov/21058170/

134. G.S. Goldman "*Vaccination to prevent varicella: Goldman and King's response to Myers' interpretation of Varicella Active Surveillance Project data*" Human and Experimental Toxicology (2014), https://www.ncbi.nlm.nih.gov/pmc/articles/PMC4363126/

135. G.S. Goldman "*Review of the United States universal varicella vaccination program: Herpes zoster incidence rates, cost-effectiveness, and vaccine efficacy based primarily on the Antelope Valley Varicella Active Surveillance Project data*"; Vaccine (2013), https://www.ncbi.nlm.nih.gov/pmc/articles/PMC3759842/pdf/main.pdf

136. Claire Dwoskin "*Merck Admits Shingles Vaccine Can Cause Eye Damage and Shingles*" The Children's Medical Safety Research Institute (2016), http://info.cmsri.org/the-driven-researcher-blog/merck-admits-shingles-vaccine-can-cause-eye-damage-and-shingles

137. Karen L. Roos "The smallpox vaccine and postvaccinal encephalitis" Seminars in Neurology (2002), https://www.ncbi.nlm.nih.gov/pubmed/?term=12170398

138. Suzanne Humphries MD "*CDC and Friends Sprinting Towards the Polio "Finish Line*" (2012), http://www.whale.to/v/cdc_and_friends.html,

139. Jim West "*Pesticides and Polio: A Critique of Scientific Literature*" The Weston A. Price Foundation (2003), https://www.westonaprice.org/health-topics/environmental-toxins/pesticides-and-polio-a-critique-of-scientific-literature/

140. Neetu Vashisht "*Polio programme: let us declare victory and move on*" Indian Journal of Medical Ethics (2012), https://pubmed.ncbi.nlm.nih.gov/22591873/

141. Rachana Dhiman "*Correlation between Non-Polio Acute Flaccid Paralysis Rates with Pulse Polio Frequency in India*" International Journal if Environmental Research and Public Health, (2018), https://www.ncbi.nlm.nih.gov/pmc/articles/PMC6121585/?report=classic

142. Yasuhiko Kubota "*Association of measles and mumps with cardiovascular disease: The Japan Collaborative Cohort (JACC) study*" Atherosclerosis (2015), https://www.ncbi.nlm.nih.gov/pubmed/26122188

143. Sebastian L. Johnston "*The protective effect of childhood infections*" British Medical Journal (2001), https://www.ncbi.nlm.nih.gov/pmc/articles/PMC1119618/

144. E. Kucukosmanoglu "*Frequency of allergic diseases following measles*"; Allergologia et Immunopathologia (2006), https://www.ncbi.nlm.nih.gov/pubmed/16854347

145. "*Top 10 pharmaceutical companies based on global vaccine revenues in 2017 and 2024*" Statista, https://www.statista.com/statistics/314562/leading-global-pharmaceutical-companies-by-vaccine-revenue/

146. "*1653 Athlete Cardiac Arrests or Serious Issues, 1148 of Them Dead, Since COVID Injection*" Good Sciencing (2023), https://goodsciencing.com/covid/athletes-suffer-cardiac-arrest-die-after-covid-shot/

147. K. Bille "*Sudden cardiac death in athletes: the Lausanne Recommendations*" European Journal of Cardiovascular Prevention and Rehabilitation (2006), https://pubmed.ncbi.nlm.nih.gov/17143117/

148. S. Mansanguan "*Cardiovascular Manifestation of the BNT162b2 mRNA COVID-19 Vaccine in Adolescents*" Tropical Medical and Infectious Journal (2022), https://pubmed.ncbi.nlm.nih.gov/36006288/

149. O. Tuvali "*The Incidence of Myocarditis and Pericarditis in Post COVID-19 Unvaccinated Patients—A Large Population-Based Study*" Journal of Clinical Medicine (2022), https://www.mdpi.com/2077-0383/11/8/2219

www.ingramcontent.com/pod-product-compliance
Ingram Content Group UK Ltd.
Pitfield, Milton Keynes, MK11 3LW, UK
UKHW021916190726
13853UKWH00002B/693

9 798887 729671